★ Reportion your plate without giving up your favorites. Discover the better alternative to a huge lunchtime sandwich.

★ Add 4½ cups of fruits and vegetables. Sounds too hard? You'll find out how to make it easy and incredibly tasty.

★ Give yourself "wiggle room"! Sugar in your coffee and a small piece of chocolate? You can!

★ Take out the bad fats. Keep in the good ones. The right amount is the key to losing weight.

★ Eat your protein *as part of a balanced* diet. You'll get clear, reliable information on the best protein sources.

★ Fiber is in! Sugar and sweeteners...not gone, but find out how much you can have.

★ Choose whole grains. They taste the best, and give nutrients that boost your immunity!

★ Count calories...but don't get blue. Your daily allowance is higher than you think (but probably less than you're consuming!)

PLUS JUST THE RIGHT AMOUNT OF EXERCISE...

THE RIGHT NUMBER OF CALORIES...

THE BEST QUALITY FOODS AND

START TO GET HEALTHIER IN JUST FOUR WEEKS!

# THE UNCLE SAM DIET

# THE
# UNCLE
# SAM
# DIET

★ The 4-Week Eating Plan ★
for a Thinner, Healthier America

Keith-Thomas Ayoob, Ed.D., R.D., FADA
and Barbara Hoffman

St. Martin's Paperbacks

# Contents

# Acknowledgments

Thanks to Tom and Diane Ayoob, who taught me the importance of food and the family. To Rod Deane, who taught me to savor it over time. To Herbert Cohen, MD, who values my work; Joan Horbiak, MPH, RD, who taught me to communicate; Barbara Baron, MS, RD, a limitless resource; my colleagues Leslie Bonci, MS, RD, David Grotto, MS, RD, and Althea Zanecosky, MS, RD, who remind me that laughter is the best nutrient; and especially to my patients and their families, who are worth everything. A special thanks to all the coffee bars that allowed me to set up my laptop on weekends and write, in exchange for buying enough fat-free, decaf lattes to float Manhattan.

Keith-Thomas Ayoob

Thanks to Phil, Marilyn, and Stephen Hoffman, who always believed—and to Bruce and Sam Locklin, who insisted. And to Faye Penn of the *New York Post*, whose big fat idea this was in the first place.

Barbara Hoffman

# THE
# UNCLE
# SAM
# DIET

# CHAPTER 1

# Stop the Diet, I Want to Get Off!

I hear you: Most diets suck (excuse the technical term). The more restrictive they are, the harder it is to stick to them. A few weeks, a few months, anyone can hack that. But then boredom and deprivation begin to sink in—and your diet sinks with them. A few "forbidden foods" later, you feel guilty about cheating, and you feel even worse when the pounds you've lost come creeping back.

But, hey, we keep hoping. Another day, another diet—and Americans have tried them all. We've low-carbed it, blood-typed it, grapefruited it, high-proteined it, zoomed right into the Zone and out of it. We've met our Maker's Diet, slept with the caveman's diet, and awakened with "Atkins breath." We've let it go with the fat-flush method and tried to burn off the calories with cider vinegar. Those of a certain age may have even hoisted a few with the drinking man's diet.

Don't forget the pills. Boy, do we love our pills. Fiber pills, mineral pills, the "scientific breakthroughs," assorted "revolutions," and the "just-take-two-of-these-before-every-meal" capsules. We've shelled out big time on "unique miracle combination" packets of supplements. None of them worked.

Remember Vacu-pants? They were these weird-looking sweatpants with a hole at the hip where you'd attach a vacuum-cleaner hose. Then you'd move around, and the jiggling stuff around your thighs would just magically melt away. Fat chance. Still, thousands of people bought them, hoping for a miracle cure and getting suckered instead.

### How fat are we?

Really fat. About six in ten adults, reports the Centers for Disease Control (CDC), are either overweight or obese. (I'll get into the technical distinction later.) The CDC makes a point of tracking these things, because most of the chronic diseases that plague Americans—heart disease, diabetes, high blood pressure, and many kinds of cancers—are more likely to strike those who weigh more than they're supposed to.

Let's put it in perspective. The most reliable source we have is telling us that more than half of us are overweight. Imagine if six in ten Americans were expected to get the flu. In most cases the flu can be prevented or endured without serious consequences. But there's no vaccine—yet—that can protect us against a chronic condition that can cause diabetes, high-blood pressure, and heart disease; take a toll on our joints; impede our breathing; slow us down; interrupt our sleep; and shorten our lives and the lives of our children.

Obesity is a significant factor in every one of those

things. Six out of ten of us are lugging around far too many more pounds than we should be. We're eating ourselves to death—and Uncle Sam has finally decided to do something about it.

### The kids are all right, right?

No, they're not. Not by a long shot. A report in the March 17, 2005, issue of *The New England Journal of Medicine* revealed that, for the first time in our history, this generation of children may have *shorter* lives than their parents. That's not just wrong—it's obscene.

The facts are these: Right now, three in ten American children are either overweight or downright obese. As a pediatric nutritionist for more than twenty years, I know. And it's heartbreaking. I'm seeing children who are prematurely old and sick—with diabetes, high blood pressure, soaring cholesterol levels, and breathing problems. They're so overweight that they can't even move around and play.

Everyone points a finger at fast food, supersizing, and TV. But it's more than that. We can help our kids—and ourselves—but we have to start now.

### Is the whole world getting fatter, or is it just America?

Good question. Truth is, we're not alone. In fact, America isn't even the fattest nation on the planet. In Greece, the country that started the Mediterranean diet craze, there is a higher percentage of obese men and women than in the United States, according to a 2005 report by the International Obesity Task Force. Cyprus, Germany, Finland, and Slovakia all have a higher percentage of overweight or obese men than the 67 percent in the United States. Even the svelte French, like so many of their European counterparts, are tipping the scales. And it would be that way even if fast food places left the Champs-Élysées.

Of course, America is still ahead of many countries—and this is one area where we don't need to lead.

### Were we always fat?

No way. In fact, we were leaner as recently as the late 1970s. Back then, only about three in twenty adults were considered obese. Now, it's twice that—six in twenty adults, according to the CDC. Just to give you some idea of how we've "grown," in the Victorian England of the 1880s, the average women's waist size was twenty-three inches. Today the average British woman's waistline is thirty inches. Here in the colonies, things aren't much better. A size eight dress size was always considered the average for women. This puts a woman's measurements at 35-27-35½. A recent national sizing study showed that seven out of ten women had hips measuring at least forty inches. Twiggy we're not. But fat isn't a feminist issue. In 1960, the average weight for men ages twenty to seventy-four was 166 pounds; by 2002 it was 191.

Are we simply eating more, or are we just eating the wrong things? The answer is a whole lotta both. We're also spending entirely too much time on our butts thinking about the next snack. It's a vicious cycle: The less we move, the less we feel like moving, and the fatter we get. So pass the chips and pop in another video.

Welcome to our big, fat American life.

**So can't we just cut out the bad foods, the way many diets tell us to do?**

Diets could work if you followed them scrupulously, but few of us can follow them forever. Most diets are restrictive and too extreme. What's the fun of having the burger if you can't have a few fries? How can you face that mountain of grains and veggies without a little olive oil? What exactly is wrong with a pat of butter on your bread once in a while?

Not long ago, a popular talk-show host weighed in (sorry) on the trials of her low-carb diet—and how, after three weeks, she craved, absolutely longed for, a green apple.

Whoa. How did a green apple suddenly become forbidden fruit? Unless we're talking about the Garden of Eden, the apple is innocent.

For that matter, there's nothing evil about potatoes, pasta, bread, rice, and (in the right quantities) chocolate. The truth is, fruits, vegetables, and whole grains are great foods—they're what we should be eating. They are not, as the gurus of low-carb diets would have you believe, the enemy. These foods won't sabotage your weight—indeed, they may help you manage it. Cutting out entire groups of foods is dangerous, especially when you drop them from your child's diet as well.

**If diets don't work, what does?**

A good eating style works, and so does an active way of life. Together, they make up what we're calling the Uncle Sam Diet. True to its name, it's liberating—not a "diet," per se, but a smarter, healthier way to live and eat.

## What do you mean by "eating style"?

An eating style is a way of life—it influences our choices and serving sizes in a way that becomes second nature. We get what we need from the foods we enjoy, and we learn to enjoy what we eat because we have such a varied selection. And in the right amounts, we can eat anything. With apologies to the diamond merchants of the world, a good eating style is forever.

A diet, by popular definition, is only temporary. Most diets, since they are short-term solutions, tend to be extreme. They exclude lots of foods, sometimes even entire food groups. There was that grapefruit diet that lasted for about ten days. The water diet that had you drinking about twelve glasses of $H_2O$ every day (with any luck, you were always a few steps from the bathroom). Then there was that cider vinegar regime where you got to eat tons of fat as long as you washed it all down with vinegar so the acid would "break up" the fat and you'd lose weight. Somebody probably made a mint on that one. How could anyone live like that? (If anything, "breaking up the fat" makes it more absorbable and more likely to stick. But don't get me started.)

Once the diet ended, the pounds returned. That's why dieting has become a gold mine—we keep regaining the same lost pounds over and over again. Some say we live to eat; others eat to live. The truth is probably somewhere in between. We weren't made for Spartan, restrictive diets. But we do need to approach food with appreciation and common sense.

Here's my rule of thumb: ANY DIET THAT MAKES ANY FOOD OFF-LIMITS IS STUPID.

Personally, I draw the line at any diet that forbids chocolate, especially the dark kind, which—in the right doses—is actually good for you. Life is hard enough without giving up the foods we love.

## So what makes up a good eating style?

It's a balance between the foods you know you need and the foods you absolutely can't live without. It should give a serious nod to health but temper it with fun and enjoyment. After all, eating is to be enjoyed and savored, even as it nourishes you.

Any eating style evolves over time. Don't expect to change your world by tomorrow. Uncle Sam wants you to go at your own pace. After all, it took Uncle Sam a while to get there, too. Take your family with you. Do it gradually, and they may not even notice.

## What kinds of eating styles work?

The kind we can stay with and grow with. Any good eating style needs to work for us and be *ours*. That means it has to be flexible. Uncle Sam knows we take things day by day. Some of us work long hours or travel a lot; others stay at home but are constantly busy. The point is, life happens. A healthy eating style is about balance, not perfection. No need to be an overachiever here.

It's also okay if you have something wicked now and then. Uncle Sam has made peace with food and encourages you to do the same. You'll find it actually enhances your life. So don't go postal: Have a slice of bread with your meal. The world won't fall in.

## What else do you need?

It's not just meals—it's motivation. In fact, it's probably more about motivation. These days, nutritionists have discovered that most people know what to do—they just have trouble getting there. Obviously, everyone is different, but here are three things we all need to get us where we want to go:

- good attitude
- persistence
- physical activity

With a good attitude, you can accept the process of gradual change. You can get over hurdles, recover from a lapse, a relapse, even a collapse in your progress.

Persistence is simply putting one foot in front of the other. When it comes to changing your eating style, slow and steady wins the race.

As for physical activity, notice I didn't say "exercise." I'll be straight up with you: If you think you can manage your health without upping your physical activity, you're kidding yourself. Trust me on this: I was such a physical zero as a kid that I was put into remedial gym class. Couldn't catch a ball if it had glue on it. Let's not even discuss throwing one. But today, I'm active and loving it because I found how to do it my way. (Cue up Sinatra.) We'll get more into physical activity in Chapter 4.

**So why eat up Uncle Sam?**

Precisely because it's *not* a diet but a better way to live. If you need to lose weight, you will—but weight isn't what this is all about. Uncle Sam puts health first. Period. That's why it's for everyone.

I work with children and adults. I know how much kids imitate their parents and how much influence parents—not peers—have on kids. Parents who eat intelligently tend to have children who do the same. Kids don't need diets. They need you.

In the next chapter, we'll get a handle on where things are for you right now.

# CHAPTER 2

# How Your Body Rates

**How do I know if I'm really overweight?**

There's a fairly easy way to tell. The most common measure is the body mass index, or BMI. It's a measure of your weight, based on your height. You want your BMI to fall between 19 and 25. Those are the normal values. Above a BMI of 25, you have two major classifications: overweight and obese.

**What's the difference between overweight and obese?**

Overweight means your BMI is at least 25 but less than 30. If your BMI is 30 or more, that's considered obese. There are also levels of obesity:

- stage I obesity: BMI = 30–34.9
- stage II obesity: BMI = 35–39.9
- stage III obesity: BMI = 40 and above

How do I figure my BMI so I know where I fall in this scheme?

Look at the table below and see where you fit in.

**Height**

| BMI | 4'10" | 4'11" | 5' | 5'1" | 5'2" | 5'3" | 5'4" | 5'5" | 5'6" | |
|-----|-------|-------|-----|------|------|------|------|------|------|---|
| 19 | 91 | 94 | 97 | 100 | 104 | 107 | 110 | 114 | 118 | |
| 20 | 96 | 99 | 102 | 106 | 109 | 113 | 116 | 120 | 124 | Healthy Weight |
| 21 | 100 | 104 | 107 | 111 | 115 | 118 | 122 | 126 | 130 | |
| 22 | 105 | 109 | 112 | 116 | 120 | 124 | 128 | 132 | 136 | |
| 23 | 110 | 114 | 118 | 122 | 126 | 130 | 134 | 138 | 142 | |
| 24 | 115 | 119 | 123 | 127 | 131 | 135 | 140 | 144 | 148 | |
| 25 | 119 | 124 | 128 | 132 | 136 | 141 | 145 | 150 | 155 | |
| 26 | 124 | 128 | 133 | 137 | 142 | 146 | 151 | 156 | 161 | |
| 27 | 129 | 133 | 138 | 143 | 147 | 152 | 157 | 162 | 167 | Overweight |
| 28 | 134 | 138 | 143 | 148 | 153 | 158 | 163 | 168 | 173 | |
| 29 | 138 | 143 | 148 | 153 | 158 | 163 | 169 | 174 | 179 | |
| 30 | 143 | 148 | 153 | 158 | 164 | 169 | 174 | 180 | 186 | |
| 31 | 148 | 153 | 158 | 164 | 169 | 175 | 180 | 186 | 192 | |
| 32 | 153 | 158 | 163 | 169 | 175 | 180 | 186 | 192 | 198 | Obese |
| 33 | 158 | 163 | 168 | 174 | 180 | 186 | 192 | 198 | 204 | |
| 34 | 162 | 168 | 174 | 180 | 186 | 191 | 197 | 204 | 210 | |
| 35 | 167 | 173 | 179 | 185 | 191 | 197 | 204 | 210 | 216 | |

**Weight in Pounds**

## Height

| BMI | 5'7" | 5'8" | 5'9" | 5'10" | 5'11" | 6' | 6'1" | 6'2" | 6'3" | |
|-----|------|------|------|-------|-------|-----|------|------|------|---|
| 19 | 121 | 125 | 128 | 132 | 136 | 140 | 144 | 148 | 152 | Healthy Weight |
| 20 | 127 | 131 | 135 | 139 | 143 | 147 | 151 | 155 | 160 | |
| 21 | 134 | 138 | 142 | 146 | 150 | 154 | 159 | 163 | 168 | |
| 22 | 140 | 144 | 149 | 153 | 157 | 162 | 166 | 171 | 176 | |
| 23 | 146 | 151 | 155 | 160 | 165 | 169 | 174 | 179 | 184 | |
| 24 | 153 | 158 | 162 | 167 | 172 | 177 | 182 | 186 | 192 | |
| 25 | 159 | 164 | 169 | 174 | 179 | 184 | 189 | 194 | 200 | Overweight |
| 26 | 166 | 171 | 176 | 181 | 186 | 191 | 197 | 202 | 208 | |
| 27 | 172 | 177 | 182 | 188 | 193 | 199 | 204 | 210 | 216 | |
| 28 | 178 | 184 | 189 | 195 | 200 | 206 | 212 | 218 | 224 | |
| 29 | 185 | 190 | 196 | 202 | 208 | 213 | 219 | 225 | 232 | |
| 30 | 191 | 197 | 203 | 209 | 215 | 221 | 227 | 233 | 240 | Obese |
| 31 | 198 | 203 | 209 | 216 | 222 | 228 | 235 | 241 | 248 | |
| 32 | 204 | 210 | 216 | 222 | 229 | 235 | 242 | 249 | 256 | |
| 33 | 211 | 216 | 223 | 229 | 236 | 242 | 250 | 256 | 264 | |
| 34 | 217 | 223 | 230 | 236 | 243 | 250 | 257 | 264 | 272 | |
| 35 | 223 | 230 | 236 | 243 | 250 | 258 | 265 | 272 | 279 | |

## Weight in Pounds

The numbers in the table are rounded off. For those Einsteins who want to figure their BMI exactly, here's the formula:

$$BMI = \frac{\text{weight in pounds}}{(\text{height in inches}) \times (\text{height in inches})} \times 703$$

Do the math. Suppose you're a 5'4" (64") woman who weighs 165 pounds. That's 165 ÷ 4,096 = 0.04 × 703 = 28.12. You're overweight—which you know from the BMI table without getting out your calculator.

Enough already with the math. What's weird is that you might not think that a guy who is 5'9" and 175 pounds would be overweight, but that's the case.

### Why aren't there different tables for men and women?

The BMI doesn't care what sex you are. There is some controversy about that, but if you're a woman, you might not want to be different, anyway. You wouldn't exactly come out ahead. The overweight numbers for women would likely start at about 24 instead of 25. So choose your battles, but women may want to choose a different one. Just let it go and look at the table.

### How do you figure BMI for kids?

The table above is for adults only. It's best to check with your child's doctor for a breakdown. There are BMI charts for kids ages two to twenty years, but it's more of a curve or a sliding scale than a set value, because they grow at different rates throughout childhood. Check with your child's pediatrician.

### BMI: the good, the bad, and the promising

The good news is that your BMI doesn't tell much about your body composition. It usually correlates pretty well for most people, but there are cases where you can be "overweight" but not "overfat" because the

BMI does not deal specifically with body composition. So if you're a bodybuilder or a pro wrestler, like The Rock, you could be bulked up with muscle, and "overweight," but still have a normal or even less than normal amount of body fat. By the way, a "normal" amount of body fat is about 15 percent for a man in his early twenties and about 23 percent for a woman of the same age. Ideally, that's where you'd like to keep it forever.

### And now the bad news

The above applies to *very* few people, and they usually know who they are. They've usually been working on their bodies for a while. That huge muscle thing doesn't just happen after a couple of bench presses on Saturday afternoon.

### But there's hope

Now that you know the "normal" BMI values, understand that it's never about being perfectly normal with Uncle Sam. It's about being better. It's about improvement. If you see improvement, fantastic. To hell with "normal" values. Look at this example:

*"I've been overweight my whole life. I'm 5 feet 9 inches and I'm supposed to weigh no more than 170 pounds. There's no way I'll ever see 170 pounds again. Does that mean I can never be healthy?"*

You can absolutely be healthier, way healthier. And feel better. If not, I wouldn't be writing this book. In fact, you can feel better and be healthier by reducing your present weight by just 10 percent. That means if you now weigh 250 pounds, losing 25 pounds and keeping it off will make a huge difference in your health. You'll also feel better, and that, as they say, is priceless.

**If 10 percent is good, isn't 20 percent better?**

Not in my book. What's not so good is to go gang-busters and lose 80 pounds to get down to 170 and then eat your way back up. Huge mistake, especially if you lose it the wrong way and too fast. I've always held that having a healthy eating style (not a "diet") *first* is.better than focusing all your attention on losing weight. The weight loss will come, and when it does, you'll be in a better position to keep it off.

**What if you have a normal BMI? Do you really need to change your eating style?**

Don't be blindsided by BMI because, as we know, it tells you only so much. I know many people who skip breakfast, eat whatever they like and as much as they like—who break every dietary rule known—and their BMI is normal, they're not overweight (don't you hate them?). They may have good intentions and want to have a better eating style, but it just doesn't work out that way. Often they see no need to change because their weight stays normal.

I'll say it again: Uncle Sam is about health, not just weight. And good health is important for everyone, no matter what their weight.

# CHAPTER 3

# Getting Down with Uncle Sam

I wish I could take the credit for it, but I didn't invent the principles of the Uncle Sam Diet. Uncle Sam's eating style is based on the principles of the 2005 Dietary Guidelines for Americans. My job is helping you decode them and make them part of your life.

In a nutshell, the guidelines are based on sound science, *all* the available sound science; get updated and revised every five years, because our knowledge of nutrition and health keeps growing; and are different this time and more specific than ever before, because we know more now about how nutrition affects our health.

No way did the feds do this stuff themselves. They brought together thirteen specialists (MDs and PhDs) to look at all the available research and think this through as a committee. Naturally, a lot of their report was printed in nutritionese. The book you're holding is your not-so-secret decoder.

What the 2005 Dietary Guidelines aren't

- They are not a prescription.
- They are not intended to cure or treat diseases. They are developed to help lower your risk and help *prevent* diseases and chronic conditions.
- They are not for people with illnesses or special nutritional needs.

---

AS ALWAYS, BEFORE STARTING ANY DIETARY CHANGES, CHECK WITH YOUR DOCTOR.

---

What the guidelines are

There's a lot to digest here, so let's make it easy. All told, the 2005 Dietary Guidelines for Americans (DGA) consist of forty-one key recommendations— twenty-three for the general public and eighteen for special populations like the elderly, children and adolescents, pregnant or lactating women, and some others. These recommendations are grouped into nine general sections:

1. Adequate nutrients within calorie needs
2. Weight management
3. Food groups to encourage
4. Fats
5. Carbohydrates
6. Sodium and potassium
7. Alcoholic beverages
8. Food safety
9. Physical activity

## ADEQUATE NUTRIENTS WITHIN CALORIE NEEDS

Guideline: *Consume a variety of nutrient-dense foods within and among the basic food groups while choosing foods that limit the intake of saturated and trans fats, cholesterol, added sugars, salt, and alcohol.*

Translation: Cut back on junk food, or what the feds kindly refer to as "foods of minimal nutritional value." Nutritionally dense foods, on the other hand, are those that give us the biggest bang for our caloric buck. These include

- grains, cereals, breads
- fruits
- vegetables
- dairy foods
- meats and meat alternatives (i.e., nuts, beans, tofu)

The second part of the guideline is pretty clear: Cut back on saturated and trans fats, cholesterol, added sugars, salt, and alcohol. This is easier than it sounds, especially if you cut back on processed foods.

Keep in mind that "limit" does not mean "eliminate." We can still include foods that have these things, but let's get real about it. The occasional pork rind is one thing. Making them your standard TV snack is another.

Guideline: *Meet recommended intakes within energy needs by adopting a balanced eating pattern, such as the US Department of Agriculture Food Guide or the*

*Dietary Approaches to Stop Hypertension (DASH) Eating Plan.*

Translation: Balance your calories in with your calories out, but do it with a good, healthy eating style.

## WEIGHT MANAGEMENT

Guideline: *To maintain body weight in a healthy range, balance calories from foods and beverages with calories expended.*

Translation: Eat what you need and no more. It's like having a "calorie bank" that relies on daily deposits and withdrawals. The government figures that the average adult needs to get about 2,000 calories per day. Many men need more than 2,000 calories, and sedentary people and women with small builds need fewer.

Of course, this calorie bank account has a cap, and if you deposit more calories into your account than it needs for the day, the overflow is transferred into the long-term savings account, also known as your body fat. No paperwork required here: The calorie bank is extremely efficient and does this automatic deposit for you. No muss, no fuss, until you get on the scale. On the flip side, if you deposit fewer calories than you need, your body taps into its long-term savings. Result: You lose some weight.

Guideline: *To prevent gradual weight gain over time, make small decreases in food and beverage calories and increase physical activity.*

Translation: This refers to that unofficial but widely known phenomenon called the "creeping five pounds syndrome." It tends to hit when you're over thirty and is often thought to be an inevitable consequence of that other widely known phenomenon called "life." What the guideline says here is that the "creeping five pounds syndrome" doesn't have to happen, but you have to stay on top of things. Above all, keep adjusting your calorie intake to meet your needs, so tweak a little here and there, and don't forget to move a little more, especially if you've been moving a little less over time.

### FOOD GROUPS TO ENCOURAGE,
### AKA "THE RIGHT STUFF"

Guideline: *Consume a sufficient amount of fruits and vegetables while staying within energy [aka calorie] needs. Two cups of fruit and 2½ cups of vegetables per day are recommended for a reference 2,000-calorie intake, with higher or lower amounts depending on the calorie level.*

Translation: Notice that it says "cups," not servings. We all know how big a cup is, while a "serving" can be anything. There were standard serving sizes, but only for the government. The rest of us never knew what they were.

So cups it is, and 4½ cups is not as much as you think. You know those pint-size plastic containers your Chinese takeout comes in? Well, save them. Each container holds 2 cups. Fill one of them with fresh fruit and you've got your quota for the day.

Same deal with vegetables, plus a little more. (If you're eating mostly raw leafy greens, which take up a lot of volume, fill yourself an additional container. Why? Remember how spinach collapses when it's cooked? That's why.) Right now the average American consumes fewer than 2 cups of fruits and vegetables a day; more often than not they're getting most of their calories from sugar and fat. By the way, the most popular "vegetable" these days? French fries.

Of course, this is all figuring that you need 2,000 calories daily. If you need fewer, you can tweak the fruits and veggies a bit, but aim for as much as you can because they're all low in calories and high in the volume you need to feel full. By the same token, if you need more than 2,000 calories, go ahead and pile on the produce.

Guideline: *Choose a variety of fruits and vegetables each day. In particular, select from all five vegetable subgroups (dark green, orange, legumes, starchy vegetables, and other vegetables) several times a week.*

Translation: This isn't a burden, it's liberation! Start with the fruit you already know and love. Think apples, oranges, pears, pineapples, watermelon, mangoes, papayas, grapefruit, nectarines, peaches, cherries, strawberries, raspberries, blueberries, plums, and grapes. (Ah, grapes, the perfect noncommitment fruit. You can take a few from the fruit bowl as you pass and move on. Or wash and freeze them, then eat as is or drop them into a glass with some juice and seltzer for a kicked-back spritzer.)

Now reach out for the more exotic stuff: Persian and crenshaw melons, lychees, kumquats, kiwis, pomegranates, Asian pears, and Sharon fruits. Don't forget dried fruits: raisins, figs, apricots, and dates.

Try to buy a new fruit each week and keep it out and open in the kitchen. Many fruits keep better at room temperature than in the fridge.

As far as vegetables go, iceberg lettuce is just . . . well, the tip of the iceberg. Think green leaf, red leaf, romaine, Boston and Bibb, plus other leafy greens: red and green Swiss chard, bok choi, chicory, dandelion, collards, kale, broccoli rabe, and cabbage of every kind and color (green, purple, Chinese, napa), and Brussels sprouts.

Take your pick of all those potatoes (white, sweet, Yukon gold, red), mind your peas and onions (brown, white, red, scallions, leeks, shallots, pearl, Vidalia, Spanish), and surround yourself with squash (summer, winter, butternut, spaghetti, pumpkin, acorn). There are too many mushroom varieties to name, but if you haven't already tried a charbroiled portobello—as meaty as a hamburger with none of the fat—time's a-wastin'.

If you like tomatoes, you'll love grape tomatoes. They're sweet as sugar and you can rinse them off in the container they come in, take them to work, and pop them into your mouth—if your coworkers don't mooch them first.

At home, wake up your plate and your palate with an array of brightly colored veggies. They're no sweat to prepare, either: baking, broiling, or grilling them concentrates flavor better than boiling. As the water goes out, the flavor stays in. Best of all, no pots to wash. Cover your oven rack with foil, bake or broil, then toss the foil for a quick cleanup.

Nearly every supermarket these days sells bags of ready-to-eat salad greens. Go easy on the dressing, and the salad days of your life will last much longer, even as you remain that much lighter.

Guideline: *Consume 3 or more ounce-equivalents of whole grain products per day, with the rest of the recommended grains coming from enriched or whole-grain products. In general, at least half the grains should come from whole grains.*

Translation: Uncle Sam finally got specific here. The old guidelines simply said "eat several servings of whole grains per day." Now we have "ounce-equivalents." I can read your mind: What in the world is that? It's the amount that would be in a 1-ounce slice of whole wheat bread. If you wanted, say, oatmeal instead, you would have ½ cup. With most ready-to-eat whole-grain cereals (Cheerios, Total, Wheaties), about 1 cup is an ounce-equivalent. So you need three of them for the day. If you mix them up, it's easy to get three over the course of a day, and it amounts to about 250 calories.

By the way, whole grain is not "bran." The whole grain means the whole package: the outer bran layer plus the germ and the endosperm (don't get excited—it simply means the white part). Each has its benefits, so figure that, in this case, the whole may just be better than the sum of its parts.

There's also room for some refined but enriched grains: the so-called white foods: most pasta, white rice, and white bread. They've been linked to everything from overweight to suicide and probably bad weather as well. But on the plus side, they're enriched with some valuable nutrients. For many kids, they're the largest source of iron. Just remember that at least half your grain intake should be from whole grain foods.

**How do I get more whole grains into my life without joining a commune?**

Hold the Birkenstocks! Whole-grain foods are mainstream now—in fact, they're everywhere. Cereals are loaded with them. Start your day with an ounce or two of typical whole grain cereals—Cheerios, Wheaties, Total, oatmeal, and Wheatina are some common ones, but there are others, so check labels. (For most dry cereals, an ounce is about a cup; for most hot cereals, it's about a half cup.) Whole grains will help you stay satisfied all morning long.

For lunch, get your sandwich on whole wheat bread or on a whole wheat pita: that gets you two servings of whole grains right there. (Bread note: Rye bread and "wheat" bread aren't all they're cracked up to be. They're okay, but they're not 100 percent whole grain. Eat them sometimes, but favor the whole-grain breads.) Ordering Chinese? Ask for brown rice. It may cost a bit more, but it's got a nice nutty taste and it will satisfy you longer than white. Make brown rice the default rice at home, too. If you want to speed up the cooking time, soak it first. Cracked wheat, better known as bulgur wheat, cooks faster than brown rice and makes a nifty substitute for white.

There are plenty of other ways to go with the grain. When you bake, use half whole wheat flour and half white—you probably won't notice the difference. If you balk at whole wheat pasta (and some people do, since it has a different texture), look for whole-grain pasta blends—regular pasta blended with whole wheat flour. You're still getting some whole grain, but the taste is more like what you know. Ditto whole wheat English muffins.

Don't forget barley—that's a whole grain, too. You can get mushroom barley soup at just about any diner. It's cheap and good for you, too.

More good news: Popcorn is a whole grain. Get an air popper and go easy on the butter. Better yet, spray with a butter-flavored popcorn spray and add all the flavor and none of the calories. It really works.


## MILKING DAIRY FOR ALL IT'S WORTH

Guideline: *Consume 3 cups per day of fat-free or low-fat milk or equivalent milk products.*

Translation: The old recommendation called for 2 to 3 "servings" (there's that word again) of milk and milk products. Now Uncle Sam is getting more specific, calling for a definite 3 cups or their equivalent: about 1½ ounces of cheese or a cup of yogurt is the same as 1 cup of milk. The accent is on the "fat-free or low-fat" choices. Why this change? Simple: The link between dairy foods, better health, and lowered risk of many chronic diseases is very strong. Indeed, the combination of dairy foods, fruits, and vegetables has been shown to lower hypertension, but there are lots of other reasons to recommend a solid consistent intake of low-fat and fat-free dairy foods.

- We need a steady supply of calcium *throughout* our lives. Milk—it's not just for kids. Most Americans don't get enough calcium, and that's bad to the bone.
- Osteoporosis is getting more common. Brittle bones aren't showing up in only women and the elderly, but in men and women in their forties and fifties.
- Kids are flunking calcium, and this is setting them up for bone problems (and maybe hypertension) later on.
- Milk is a protein drink. It has, along with eggs, the highest quality protein you can get.
- Milk is one of the few dietary sources of vitamin D, which helps you absorb and process calcium.
- If you don't eat dairy foods, chances are you're not getting the calcium you need.
- Beyond protein and calcium, milk has a terrific nutrient package: 17 nutrients in total, and without a lot of calories. Now *that*'s nutrient density.

Think of low-fat and fat-free dairy foods as great vehicles for other foods we want to encourage: milk goes great with whole-grain cereal, yogurt is perfect with fresh fruit, even cheese has its place; just try to go easy on cheese and keep it to about 3 or 4 ounces per week.

**How do I get 3 cups of milk a day without turning into a dairy queen?**

Easy. Upgrade your coffee break and take a nonfat latte vacation. Two lattes a day keep bone fractures at bay.

At home, try fat-free milk powder in your coffee. Stop wincing. It's got loads of protein and calcium, and you can add as much as you want and it won't cool your coffee.

Alternatively, try fat-free evaporated milk. It's double-strength, so you'll get more bang for the drop. Since it's already liquid, you don't have to wait for it to dissolve.

Another great source of dairy is low-fat cheese. (Forget fat-free cheese. Have it if you like, but I think it's a travesty.) Low-fat cheese has come a long way. About 1½ ounces is roughly equivalent to a cup of milk.

Still, it's hard to give up the sheer sensual pleasure of full-fat cheeses like Brie and Camembert. Treat yourself to about 3–4 ounces of full-fat cheese per week. Light yogurt has come of age. It has less sugar than regular and tastes like dessert. Add it to smoothies, dip your fruit into it, and stir granola or oatmeal into it for a quick breakfast or afternoon snack. You can even top baked potatoes with plain yogurt or shredded low-fat cheese for extra calcium.

Making pancakes? Add milk powder, yogurt, or nonfat milk to the batter for a calcium boost.

There's always room for sugar-free gelatin. Make it

with half water and half milk. A generous one cup serving is another 4 ounces of milk.

The Uncle Sam menus use small amounts of grated Parmesan cheese. Even a teaspoon added to salads or sprinkled over veggies or rice will up your dairy quotient for the day—with very few calories.

Put shredded low-fat cheese on veggies or stir it into rice. It doesn't take much. A quarter cup will do for a few servings, and that's only an ounce.

## THE FATS OF LIFE

Guideline: *Keep total fat intake between 20 to 35 percent of calories, with most fats coming from sources of polyunsaturated and monounsaturated fatty acids, such as fish, nuts, and vegetable oils.*

Translation: This doesn't necessarily mean a low fat diet. It means you have options. Low to moderate fat is just fine, but the type of fat is just as important as how much. The aim used to be to keep total fat to 30 percent or less of calories. No more. Now Uncle Sam is flexible. Low-fat diets, moderate-fat diets—they can both be good.

**What does 20 or 35 percent of your calories look like?**

Well, 20 percent is easy to picture, because it's not much. In a 2,000-calorie diet, that's about 400 calories. That might sound like a lot, but it isn't. An ounce of almonds (about 24) has about 170 calories, of which about 140 are from fat. Figure that even a 4-ounce boneless, skinless chicken breast has about 90 fat calories. On a 20 percent fat diet, eat just those two foods, and you'll have consumed more than half your fat quota for the day. Here's the payoff: By eating so little fat, you're more likely to eat many more fruits, vegetables, whole grains, and fat-free dairy foods. Along the way, you'll be getting lots more fiber and reduce your risk of heart disease.

Not surprisingly, many people are either unable or unwilling to make such a drastic cut in fat. It can be a hard diet to stay on for the long term.

If that's the case, Uncle Sam says you can safely get 35 percent of your daily 2,000 calories from fat. That would give you 700 fat calories to play with each day, and you can eat well on that.

But don't go whole hog. Do salmon more often than fatty ribs. Think almonds and olive oil more than pork rinds and Crisco. That way, you can have that nice vinaigrette on your salad, and you can munch on those almonds. Remember that you still have the same 2,000 calories to play around with. Having some fat in your diet means you'll eat a bit less volume than with the lower fat diets, but for many, that's fine because they like the flavor, and flavor counts. It also allows you a little more flexibility when you eat out and when you socialize.

**Aren't some fats better than others?**

Short answer, yes. All fats are loaded with calories, but monounsaturated and polyunsaturated fats are better for your heart. Basically, these are fats that are liquid at room temperature, like olive oil and vegetable oils.

Most whole foods have a mix (few things are 100 percent in nature), but the fats in vegetable oils like olive, canola, and soybean, and in nuts like almonds and peanuts are also loaded with mono and poly fats. The same goes for most of the fat in fish, even the fatty ones. The total amount of fat in your diet is also important. Of course, you can have too much of a good thing. Nuts are great, as long as you keep portions reasonable—about an ounce or an ounce and a half a day. What's an ounce? It fills an empty Velamints tin. An ounce and a half fills an empty Altoids container (now you know what to do with all those empty breath mint boxes!).

Too much saturated fat raises your level of "bad" cholesterol and your risk of heart disease. Still, it's hard to cut out saturated fats completely, and there's no need to. Luckily, we've got many low-fat variations of our favorite foods to choose from, which is kind of like eating your cake and having it, too.

### A fish story (with nuts)

Uncle Sam wants us to get some of our fat from fish. That's because they're high in omega-3 fats, alias "good-guy fats." The main ones are called DHA and EPA for short (don't ask). These are terrific because if you eat them regularly, they can lower the consequences of heart disease (aka death). ALA (alpha-linoleic acid) is another omega-3 fatty acid that's also a player that's good for heart health; it's found mostly in walnuts, flaxseed, and to a lesser extent soybean oil.

Which fish are highest in these good fats?

Fatty fish, big time. Think salmon, herring, mackerel, and sardines. Try having a 3- or 4-ounce portion about twice a week. (That's the size of a deck of cards or a computer mouse.) Anyone who has had a "cardiac event" or some form of heart disease should eat even more fish. Leaner fish like cod, sole, and halibut have smaller amounts of omega-3 fats, so they don't really count as a "fatty fish," but they're still good because they are naturally low in calories.

What about all the noise about chemicals in fish?

The main chemicals cited as a concern are mercury and PCBs. A few fish and shellfish have more mercury than others. Why the fuss? Because excessive mercury can damage a developing fetus or a young child's central nervous system. Tuna and bluefish are cited often as being especially high in mercury—not enough for the government to advise against eating them, but they do warn young children and women who are pregnant or who might become pregnant to limit their consumption of these and other fish high in mercury. The Food and Drug Administration has a great information hotline on the latest info about warnings on fish and mercury: (www.cfsan.fda.gov/~dms/admehg3/html, or you can call 1-800-SAFEFOOD [1-800-723-3366]).

As far as PCBs go, most of the attention has been on salmon, especially farmed salmon, the kind most of us can afford. These days it's hard to find wild salmon most of the year. Some markets even pass off farmed as wild, because they look the same. A study in the journal *Science* showed that farmed salmon has more of these PCBs than wild. Great. We're supposed to eat more fish, more fatty fish, and the one we like best and can afford has those PCBs. My family has loved and eaten salmon for years—my grandfather fished it out of the San Francisco Bay—but now that it's mostly farmed, I did some investigating.

And what did you find, Sherlock? We're doomed, right?

Wrong. Salmon, including farmed salmon, is safe to eat. Here's why.

The PCBs in salmon come from fish meal, which is made up of ground up fish and edible plants. To lower the PCBs in farmed salmon, you need only reduce the amount in their feed. That's what the farmed salmon industry did, and it did the trick. Unfortunately, the *Science* study used old data that didn't reflect the new dietary formulation and the even lower PCB level.

Here's the shocker: Ounce for ounce, roast chicken has higher levels of PCBs than farmed salmon. You read that right. Meat loaf is about on par with salmon. No one is concerned about roast chicken or meat loaf, nor should they be. The PCB levels in these foods are so low as to be inconsequential. You're placing yourself at far greater risk by avoiding eating salmon than by eating it and other fish more regularly. Remove the skin from the salmon and the PCB content falls even farther. Remember, the studies that found positive health properties from eating fatty fish like salmon used the same types of fatty fish that are available to us. The researchers shopped where we shop, after all.

Guideline: *Consume less than 10 percent of calories from saturated fatty acids and less than 300 mg/day of cholesterol, and keep trans fatty acid consumption as low as possible.*

Translation: This is mostly about heart health. Saturated fat and trans fat tend to raise your "bad" LDL cholesterol." Uncle Sam says that, on a 2,000-calorie diet, eat no more than 200 calories of saturated fat. Here's what that would look like at different calorie levels.

| Total calories per day | Keep daily saturated fat to a maximum of |
|---|---|
| 1,600 | 18 grams |
| 2,000 | 22 grams |
| 2,200 | 24 grams |
| 2,500 | 28 grams |
| 2,800 | 31 grams |

Roughly half of the saturated fat we eat comes from animal sources, but plants are a source also. That's because in nature, fats tend to be found in combinations. No food has *only* monounsaturated fats or *only* saturated fat. Vegetable fats that have lots of saturated fat are the following:

- coconut oil
- palm oil
- palm kernel oil

These fats actually have more saturated fat than many animal fats, so you want to eat less of them.

Since most of our saturated fat still comes from animal foods, getting lean and mean with your butcher might be a good idea. Go skinless for sure. Take it off, take it all off. But you don't have to give up red meat. There are nineteen cuts of beef that have less fat, ounce per ounce, than skinless, boneless chicken thighs. These include top sirloin, flank steak, rib steak, bottom round, and 95 percent lean ground beef. And eye round is nearly neck and neck with skinless, boneless chicken breast. So to all you carnivores, let not your hearts be troubled. Uncle Sam gets it.

Another lean option is pork, if you trim the visible fat, but, as with beef, size definitely matters. So rein in those steakhouse excursions, and if you do visit, skip the pound of porterhouse and the bucket of mashed potatoes. And plan on taking some of that meat home. Instead, go for the lean but tasty cuts like flank and skirt steaks. Trust me, you'll feel better the next day, when you don't have to let your belt out another notch.

### What exactly is trans fat?

It starts out as liquid fat, usually a vegetable oil, but turns hard through processing. This makes it more desirable to food processors because it's way cheaper than butter and helps muffins, cookies, and cakes stay moist without leaking oil when they cool. (Hey, appearance is everything.)

You can check out which foods have trans fat by reading the nutrition facts label.

**I use margarine instead of butter. Which is better?**

Most margarines have some trans fat. A good rule of
thumb: the softer the better. Tub margarine has less
trans fat than stick margarine, and those liquid
squeeze-bottle margarines have even more polyunsaturated fat and less trans fat, if any. There are also some
tub margarines now that have no trans fats at all, so
check the nutrition facts panel on the package. Butter
has more saturated fat. It also has a little trans fat, but
it's a natural trans fat, which is different chemically
from the stuff in margarine, and natural trans fat may
even have some benefits. So a little butter on your corn
or potato is fine—just balance it by skipping the cheese
that day.

**What are the main sources of trans fat in our diet?**

These are the trans fat culprits, the worst listed first:

- cake, cookies, and baked goods
- meat and dairy fats
- margarine
- fried potatoes (and anything else that is deep-
  fried)
- chips and popcorn (packaged or movie theater
  variety)
- shortening (i.e., Crisco)

If you want to lose weight, these are foods you
should be eating in moderation anyway.

## What about cholesterol?

Uncle Sam says don't exceed 300 milligrams per day. That's the amount in about 9 ounces of cooked bacon, or a third of a pound of shrimp, or an egg and a half, or 14 ounces of ground beef, no matter if it's 95 percent lean or only 70 percent lean (that's not too lean, by the way). But 300 milligrams per day is just an average: You may be over on some days and under on others. If you do adhere to this limit, you'll naturally be limiting your consumption of most fatty meats and a good portion of saturated fat. That's because in nature, cholesterol often hangs out with saturated fat. Not always, though. Cholesterol and saturated fats have some different interests. Tropical oils like coconut and palm oil are high in saturated fat but have no cholesterol, while eggs and shellfish are high in cholesterol but low in saturated fat.

It's an important distinction because, when it comes to raising the cholesterol level in our blood (and risk of heart disease), *saturated fat* is the main culprit. Cholesterol, by itself, is a minor player. Even the American Heart Association, after a number of years, has found no evidence that limiting eggs lowers your cholesterol level. I agree with the American Heart Association on this one. Bottom line, watch your saturated fat. Don't worry as much about cholesterol, especially if it's coming from eggs or shellfish.

Eggs are a terrific nutrient package. Their protein quality is tops—the best, in fact. Eggs are also inexpensive, fast to prepare, easy to chew, and versatile. They are even one of the few dietary sources of vitamin D. Yet people got one message about eggs years

ago and didn't listen to anything else. I've actually had
adults in my office who care for very ill, emaciated
children with HIV who reassured me, "but I don't give
him eggs," fearing that they would harm his health.
Nothing could be farther from the truth.

Of course, there's plenty in eggs for the rest of us,
too. Lutein and zeaxanthin may help prevent age-
related macular degeneration, a leading cause of blind-
ness in the elderly. So don't diss eggs. Nutritionally
they're all they're cracked up to be.

> **Dr. Keith's recommendation:** The American Heart
> Association no longer has restrictions on eggs. But let's be
> smart about it. Skip the sausage and have some fresh fruit
> and whole-grain toast with your eggs instead. Have a veg-
> gie omelet instead of one with bacon. And try "frying" your
> eggs with non-stick cooking spray or a touch of olive oil
> instead of butter.

As for shellfish, the same rule applies: Keep it real.
Shellfish are low in fat, so they're great when you're
counting calories. Indeed, if you order shellfish in a
restaurant, you can be almost assured that your portion
size will be modest. Just look for them broiled, baked,
or steamed—not fried.

## The meat of the matter

Uncle Sam isn't necessarily a vegetarian, although you
can be one if you like and still follow the Uncle Sam
Diet. For omnivores, figure about 6 ounces of meat per
day, or the equivalent. That's not huge, but your plate

will still be full. The traditional "meat" food group actually includes a whole lot of other foods: lean beef for sure, but also eggs, fish (especially fatty fish), and beans and nuts. Here are some tips for getting all you can from this nutrient-rich food group:

- Get the leanest meat you can find. Ground beef should be at least 90 percent lean—95 percent is even better.
- Try ground turkey instead of fatty ground beef. It's often cheaper, too.
- Beef up your ground round with "crumbles"— the soy protein that looks and tastes like ground beef but has less fat and more protein. Mix half and half, and you're the only one who knows it.
- Turn toward tofu. Dice and mix *firm* tofu into sauces and soups to weave in some healthy protein with no extra cooking. Great in pasta sauce!
- Take the pinto out for a spin—and drive it into some good lean chili. Keep cans of different beans around. Rinse well and you'll lose about 40 percent of the sodium! Throw beans into a salad. Better yet, make a multibean salad. Good olive oil and vinegar and some grated Parmesan bring it all together.
- Get more mileage from your leftovers. Shred and use the meat from that solitary chicken drumstick or tail end of the roast to turn a pot of vegetable soup into a meal (even a winter breakfast).
- Lay an egg—over your leftovers. Figure one or two per person when you scramble them with

leftover shredded meat, potatoes, pasta, beans, whatever you have lying around the fridge.

**A final word on fat**

The "20 to 35 percent of calories" recommendation needs tweaking when it comes to children and adolescents. Their needs are different at certain stages of development. Thirty-five percent of calories from fat is still the upper limit, but the guidelines recommend that children two to three years of age get at least 30 percent of their calories from fat; adolescents should keep at least 25 percent of their calories as fat.

## THOSE CRAZY CARBS!

I *love* carbohydrates. We're just now starting to emerge from carbophobia. Carbs have been demonized for years, but we're finally recognizing them for what they are:

- Carbs are the basis of most of the world's diet.
- Foods high in carbs can be *loaded* with nutrition.
- Even refined carbs (white food) can be included when you eat with Uncle Sam.
- Most of the world uses carbs as the staple of their diet.

There's been a huge study on carbs that's been going on for centuries and shows that having carbs as the basis for your diet does not make you fat. That huge study is called Asia. As in the continent. That's right. Many cultures eat rice for breakfast, lunch, and dinner. And don't even think of taking pasta away from Italians, or baguettes from the French.

Here's what Uncle Sam has to say about carbs:

Guideline: *Choose fiber-rich fruits, vegetables, and whole grains often.*

**How often—and how many calories will that cost me?**

The actual amount will vary somewhat, based on the specific foods you choose. And it'll still leave you with room for a few wicked pleasures, like ice cream and chocolate. Assuming you mix it up, you'll average the following:

| | |
|---|---|
| 2 cups of fruits | 240 calories |
| 2½ cups of vegetables | 125 calories |
| 3 one-ounce equivalents of whole grains | 240 calories |
| Total fruits, veggies, whole grains: | 605 calories |

Not bad. That's less than one-third of your calories for the day, but look at the volume! Of course, the calories can range anywhere from about 425 calories if you choose your fruits and veggies as mostly melon and salad greens, to 850 calories if you focus more on bananas and apples and potatoes.

Of course, you'd get more calories in there if you fried those veggies or added butter to them, but you won't need to once you learn to flavor your foods without adding as much fat. Salsa on a baked potato or some intense pasta sauce on broccoli can make you forget all about butter and hollandaise sauce.

**Fiber-rich fruits and veggies? How much "fiber" are we talking about here?**

The recommendation is 14 grams per 1,000 calories. Here's what that looks like:

| Daily calories | Daily fiber (grams) |
|:---:|:---:|
| 1,400 | 20 |
| 1,600 | 22 |
| 1,800 | 25 |
| 2,000 | 28 |
| 2,200 | 31 |
| 2,400 | 34 |
| 2,600 | 36 |
| 2,800 | 39 |
| 3,000 | 42 |

The average adult gets only about 10–15 grams of fiber daily, only half as much as we need.

Truth is, when you talk about fiber, most people think constipation. Let's move past those memories of Grandpa and his stewed prunes and see what else fiber can do.

Fiber lowers your risk of heart disease and your chances of getting type 2 diabetes. If you are diabetic, fiber helps manage your blood sugar. And of course, fiber keeps you regular, as Grandpa used to say.

**What foods are the best sources of fiber? Do I have to eat hay?**

Fruits, vegetables, whole grain (including whole-grain breads and cereals), and beans. Ah, the lowly bean—so abused and yet so good for you. Introduce beans gradually into your diet and you won't suffer their most dreaded side effect. Or, as Mel Brooks immortalized them in *Blazing Saddles*: "beans, beans, the magical fruit, the more you eat, the more you toot."

Sorry, Mel, but they really are great for you. And there are so many of them: kidney beans (chili), garbanzos (hummus, anyone?), reds, whites, pinks, field beans, black-eyed peas, pea beans, lentils, split peas, and the list goes on and on. They're loaded with fiber and a whole lot of nutrition. They blend with all kinds of dishes, and you can add them to just about anything on your plate. So they're a really easy way to kick up the fiber grams. Aim for some kind of beans several times each week.

**How much fiber do beans have compared to other foods?**

Check it out:

- ½ cup lentils or split peas: 5–9 grams
- ½ cup berries: 3–4 grams
- ½ cup cooked vegetables: 2–4 grams
- 1 slice white bread: 1 gram

By adding just a half cup of beans to your day, you can get a lot closer to the fiber guideline. Just go gradually, so you and your digestive tract can make the change together, without clearing out a room.

Now throw that laxative away and have an apple.

**Speaking of apples, what about fruit juice? That's a natural carb, no?**

Sure, it's natural, and juice is fine—up to a point: one cup per day. Sure, it counts as part of your fruit consumption, but there are things in whole fruits that never make it into the juice. Like fiber.

**What if I make my own juice in a juicer and put in all kinds of fruits and veggies? Is that any better?**

You're still better off doing the whole fruit and vegetable thing. Your gut is a juicer—it just works more slowly! And that's okay. It's the way it's supposed to be. I've had patients who use their juicers faithfully. I ask them what they do with the pulp and they say, "I throw it away." But the pulp is the best part. And having the whole fruit gives you the satisfaction that comes with chewing. Chewing takes more time, as opposed to swigging down a glass of juice, so you're more likely to feel full with the same (or fewer) calories.

Note for children: The American Academy of Pediatrics says, and I absolutely agree, to limit young children to 4 to 6 ounces of juice daily, and older children and adolescents to 8 to 12 ounces daily. After that, it's the whole fruit.

**Dr. Keith on kids:** Parents tell me all the time that their kids like lots of different fruits and veggies. Then I take a diet history, and I see little or no fruits or veggies. Put back their *favorite* fruits and vegetables. Keep them around *all the time.* Make them part of meals and snacks. It's a win-win. They like them, so no food fights, and they get healthier (and you get happier).

Guideline: *Choose and prepare foods and beverages with little added sugars or caloric sweeteners.*

Translation: In the 2,000-calorie diet, figure on about 200 "discretionary calories." What do we mean by discretionary calories? Think of them as caloric mad money, to spend as you see fit. Uncle Sam figures that will be about 2 tablespoons of all kinds of added fats (about 18 grams) or about 4 tablespoons of sugars, syrups, etc., or any combination thereof. The point is that it's not a lot of calories, especially when you realize that so many fats and sugars are added to our food.

Here are where most of our added sugars are coming from:

- Soft drinks, fruit drinks and ades, including powdered drink mixes (these give us 40 percent of our added sugars!)
- candy
- cake, cookies, other pastry
- sweetened dairy

**How much soda do we drink every day?**

The average American drinks about 18 ounces daily. That's about a can and a half of regular soda! That's too much, for two reasons:

- These are empty calories. No nutrition here.
- These calories are easily replaced with sugar-free, calorie-free alternatives.

Remember, this is just the average. We all know people who consume lots more. Adolescents have come into my office lugging 1-liter bottles of soda. Not surprisingly, they tend to be my more overweight patients. The problem is that we have come to think of these amounts as normal portions, and they most definitely are not.

Bottom line: you have about 200–250 "discretionary calories" each day on a 2,000 calorie diet. If you are cutting calories to lose weight, you can still have some of these "mad money" calories—say, about 10 percent of your total. So on a diet of about 1,500 calories, that's about 150 discretionary calories, which happens to be enough for an ounce of dark chocolate! I told you I've got your back.

## SODIUM AND POTASSIUM

Sodium is just half of table salt (aka sodium chloride). The more sodium in your diet, the greater the risk of high blood pressure. High blood pressure raises your risk of heart disease, stroke, and kidney disease. It also raises the likelihood of your doctor putting you on a really restrictive diet that's not so fun.

**How much sodium are most people getting now?**

About 4,500 milligrams. That's the amount in about 2 measuring teaspoons of table salt.

**How much *should* we be getting?**

Guideline: *Consume less than 2,300 mg of sodium per day. Choose and prepare foods with little salt. At the same time, eat potassium-rich foods such as fruits and vegetables.*

But maybe you never add salt at the table. Do you still need to cut back on salt? Probably. More than 75 percent of our sodium comes from processed foods.

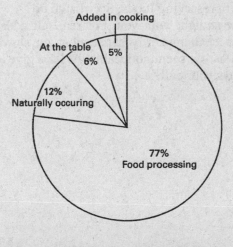

Added in cooking

At the table
6%

5%

12%
Naturally occuring

77%
Food processing

**HOW WE GET OUR SODIUM**

Source: Mattes RD, Donnelly D. Relative contributions of dietary sodium sources. *J Am Coll Nutr.* 1991 Aug; 10 (4) : 383–93.

You don't have to eat a lot of junk food to get a lot of sodium. Almost any canned or packaged food has added sodium. Not just chips and pretzels and obviously salty snacks like those. These foods also have lots of sodium:

- soups (canned and dry-packaged)
- tomato sauce
- cured meats
- canned vegetables
- condiments (soy sauce, mustard, ketchup, steak sauce, and so on)
- seasoned salt (garlic salt, onion salt, and others)
- frozen dinners

Salt is added for taste, and it's one of the oldest means of preserving foods. So what to do?

I'll be straight with you. For real salt addicts, this can be a challenge. My suggestion: go slowly. That way it'll hardly seem noticeable. At least give it a shot. It's always your call.

**Licking the salt craving—one man's saga:** Let's call him Joey. His doctor referred him to me after prescribing a low-sodium diet to manage Joey's rocket-high blood pressure. Joey was a salt addict. He loved chips of all kinds, along with Italian food and fries. He worshipped Chinese food, cold cuts, and ham. Joey's diet was a virtual festival of sodium. This man prayed to the sodium god and feared that his culinary life as he knew it would be over. Nevertheless, he cut way down on salty foods (even more than I said was necessary). After a week, Joey complained, "Doc, nothing has any taste." Such are the hazards of going cold turkey. So he moderated a bit, and when he came to see me after about six weeks, he was a happy camper. "Things taste way better now. But I bit into a hot dog the other day and I couldn't believe how salty it tasted. I don't remember it being that salty." Way to go, Joey. Your taste buds have arrived.

The point is that our taste buds change. Slow, gradual changes are unnoticeable. Think I'm kidding? Well, I can tell you that a very popular soup company, one that you probably grew up with, has gradually been lowering the sodium in its canned soups for years. Nobody noticed.

Good news: Just cut back some on processed foods and watch your sodium intake drop like a bomb. There are now tons of "no-salt-added" substitutes for most high-salt canned foods, like tomato sauce and tuna. There's even a reduced-sodium soy sauce. With Uncle Sam's new guidelines, stand back and watch more companies lowering the salt in their products.

A bonus: As you cut back on sodium, you'll wake up your sleepy taste buds. You'll have a much more sophisticated palate and will be able to notice more subtle flavors in foods. Herbs and spices will matter more because the sodium cloud will have lifted a bit. You'll find that food tastes fresher, not slaughtered.

Sigh of relief: We're not talking sodium-free here. You'll still be getting plenty of salt and sodium, but you'll be able to use it more discriminatingly and only when you find it really necessary.

---

**Little hint for happy living:** I find that I like my scrambled eggs with just a dash of salt. Sometimes I use Tabasco sauce instead—it adds almost no sodium but a truckload of flavor. As for canned chicken broth, get the reduced-sodium kind or use one part regular and one part low-sodium in cooking. Cooking things like soups and stews a day or two in advance *really* helps you add less sodium. The flavors marry and intensify over time. That's why these kinds of dishes are "better the second day." Also, don't forget lemon juice as a flavor enhancer, just like salt. A good squeeze into the pot or on your broccoli and you can get by with a lot less salt. Another great flavor enhancer is grated Parmesan cheese. It has some salt, but add just a teaspoon to your tossed salad or to potatoes or rice, you won't believe the results. It also means you can bypass some of the salty salad dressings out there and go for some good olive oil and balsamic vinegar instead.

---

## What's up with potassium?

It helps reduce high blood pressure, it holds back some of the effects of salt on your blood pressure, and it can even help reduce bone loss in older people.

## How much potassium do you need?

The short answer: Eat your 4½ cups of fruits and veggies, and get 3 servings of low-fat dairy, and forget about it—it's done. For those who want numbers, aim for 4,700 milligrams daily. Children ages one to three years should get about 3,000 milligrams of potassium each day, while those ages three to eight need 3,800, and ages nine to thirteen need 4,500 milligrams daily.

## Does this mean lots of bananas and OJ?

Expand your horizons. *All* fruits and vegetables have potassium. Citrus fruits and berries are loaded with it. So are all the leafy greens and tomatoes. And hail the mighty potato. White or sweet, red or russet, potatoes are loaded with potassium. Chips are okay occasionally (ever try plantain chips?), and make your own oven fries. Check out the recipe on page 165 and get those taters back on your plate.

## DRINKING WITH UNCLE SAM

The 2005 Dietary Guidelines acknowledge that Prohibition is a thing of the past. Americans drink, though slightly fewer of us are drinking these days. As of 2002, about 45 percent considered themselves teetotalers, compared with only 35 percent five years earlier.

Some drinking can actually be a good thing. Research shows that moderate alcohol consumption can lower your risk of death from coronary heart disease.

This is a touchy subject, because any time the feds praise alcohol consumption, some people use it as an excuse to drink themselves silly. Here's the new government line about alcohol:

Guideline: *Those who drink alcoholic beverages should do so sensibly and in moderation—defined as the consumption of up to one drink per day for women and up to two drinks per day for men.*

Translation: This was perhaps the most carefully worded recommendation of all. Note that it begins, "Those who drink alcoholic beverages . . ." This doesn't mean that people should drink, only that if they choose to do so, there's a right way to do it ("sensibly and in moderation") and a really, really wrong way to do it (anything else).

The feds have their own idea of moderation and it may be different from yours, but theirs has science behind it, so it wins. As far as the seeming sexism goes, men get to drink more because men tend to be larger than women and have a better ability to metabolize the booze. It has nothing to do with who gets drunk faster.

If you drink with Uncle Sam, you'll be healthy, not hammered.

What exactly is "one drink"?

Glad you asked. The government defined that, too. One drink is equal to any one of the following:

- 12-ounce bottle/can of regular beer
- 5-ounce glass of wine (red or white)

- 1½ ounces of 80-proof liquor (gin, vodka, bourbon, etc.)
- 3 ounces of sweet dessert-type wine (port, sherry, etc.)

These amounts may not be what you're used to getting from your favorite bartender, or what you're pouring for yourself at home. Beer is easy to measure—it usually comes in 12-ounce cans and bottles.

Five ounces of wine is probably less than you're used to seeing in a glass, especially if you drink from those globe-type glasses. It's amazing how much those seemingly modest-size goblets can hold. At any rate, it's worth finding out how much your favorite wine glass at home holds, so stop the madness and just go and measure 5 ounces of water (½ or an 8-ounce measuring cup, plus 2 tablespoons) and see how much of that glass it really fills. This will be a real eye-opener. Some of those goblets can hold more than 16 ounces. Forewarned is forearmed.

**Fine, but how do I figure this out when I'm in a restaurant?**

There is an easy way to estimate. The average bottle of wine holds about 25 ounces. That means that it should deliver five glasses, or "servings," of wine. In theory, that means that five women at lunch or dinner need to order only one bottle of wine for the entire table. No kidding. According to the feds, that's moderation for women. The same bottle could alternatively be divided by two men and a woman, or three women and a man. You get the idea. And that assumes that there has been no aperitif, no apple martini, no gin and tonic, no cosmo, etc. The point here is that it really doesn't take a heck of a lot of booze to "drink moderately," so budget accordingly.

If this news hasn't taken some of the wind from your sails yet, then I'll put in my own two cents. This comes from me, not the feds, but I'm sure they'd agree with me. With other aspects of the Uncle Sam Diet, it's about averaging your consumption over time—say, a week or two. *With alcohol, this rule does not apply.* It's one or two drinks daily, use 'em or lose 'em. No averaging out over time. No abstaining all week and saving it all up for the big blast on Saturday. Sorry, Charlie.

**The good news: You can have a drink every day**

That might make the change to smaller quantities easier. Uncle Sam isn't pushing Prohibition. Enjoy that glass of wine once a day if you like. If you live to tie one on every weekend, you may need the help and support that are out there for you. Investigate them.

---

**Dr. Keith's digression:** Uncle Sam has really defined moderation in drinking. It's probably the one place in the health arena where moderation is clearly stated. Nutritionists often speak about a diet that includes favorite foods "in moderation" but that term is seldom defined, and that confuses even the experts. After all, what good is telling consumers to eat in moderation if no one can even define moderation? Vague doesn't work for me. But when it comes to health issues, sometimes vague is all you can do, because the science just isn't there to allow more specifics. With alcohol, things are clear. This is not to say that you *can't* have more than one or two drinks, just that more than two drinks a day may be setting you up for a fall.

Of course, in terms of managing weight, there are some very good reasons for limiting your consumption to one or two drinks per day.

Give me one

Here are two. First, alcohol has calories. Sometimes a lot of them. Check out the table.

| Drink | Calories per ounce | Typical serving (ounces) | Calories per serving |
|---|---|---|---|
| Beer (regular) | 12 | 12 | 144 |
| Beer (light) | 9 | 12 | 108 |
| Wine (white) | 20 | 5 | 100 |
| Wine (red) | 21 | 5 | 105 |
| Wine (dessert) | 47 | 3 | 141 |
| Distilled spirits (40% alcohol— 80 proof) | 64 | 1½ | 96 |

Source: Agricultural Research Service Nutrient Database for Standard Reference (SR), Release 17.

So swig down that single drink of vodka on the rocks, and you'll have nearly 100 calories. Add 6 ounces of grapefruit juice (that's called a greyhound), and you can add another 90 calories, for a total of about 190 calories for that drink. Replacing the juice with soda would give you about as much, with none of the potassium or vitamin C of the juice. (This is hardly the way to get your daily quota of fruit, guys.)

See how several drinks can add up? If you're consuming 2,000 calories per day, then one drink gives you almost 10 percent of your daily calories but not a lot of nutrients to go with them. But we digress.

The other reason to keep the drinking to a minimum is more subtle. Alcohol is a "disinhibitor," meaning that after hoisting a few, you're less likely to care about making sound judgments about what and how much you'll eat. It doesn't mean you're hammered. You may be able to have a normal conversation and such, but you're also more likely to say, "Eh, that looks good. Yeah, bring it on, let's live a little." Ask anyone who has counseled substance users of any kind, and he'll tell you that alcohol and making sound judgments, or doing any other task, for that matter, don't mix.

Remember, the idea of good eating and a healthy lifestyle is to have what you like but keep it real, and you'll keep enjoying it for a long time.

Another plus: waking up the next morning able to enjoy the day, rather than recovering from the night before. You'll also be able to manage your weight better, having spared yourself all those extra empty calories—and a whole other kind of headache.

Guideline: *Alcoholic beverages should not be consumed by some individuals, including those who cannot restrict their alcohol intake, women of childbearing age who may become pregnant, pregnant and lactating women, children and adolescents, individuals taking medications that can interact with alcohol, and those with specific medical conditions.*

Translation: Alcohol isn't for everyone, regardless of any possible health benefits it may have.

If you can't seem to stop once you get going, don't start. Period. If you "have to have a drink," you probably shouldn't.

If you're planning to conceive, or are pregnant or nursing, don't drink. I have seen too many patients whose mothers drank when they were pregnant. These are the victims of fetal alcohol syndrome, children born with serious learning and behavioral problems that could have been avoided. Nine months of teetotaling (and several more if you breast-feed) will pay you back every time you look at your healthy baby.

When it comes to children and adolescents and alcohol, Uncle Sam says no.

**But look at France, where children routinely get a little wine with dinner**

It's true—many Mediterranean cultures do let children drink at the dinner table. I got a little wine at home once in a while when I was growing up.

The problem with this is that it's extremely easy to see this practice going wild. I was lucky. I had parents who practiced true moderation. They never got drunk, even at home. I saw only reasonable drinking practices. Not everyone is that lucky, and besides, there is a huge health case against giving booze to growing bodies. All in all, it's not recommended.

Guideline: *Anyone taking medications that can interact with alcohol should abstain.*

There are tons of medications that don't mix with alcohol—too many to list here, so ALWAYS ask your physician and pharmacist if you're taking medications.

> Guideline: *Alcoholic beverages should be avoided by individuals engaging in activities that require attention, skill, or coordination, such as driving or operating machinery.*

These are no-brainers. Even over-the-counter medications may not mix with alcohol, so *always* read the label. Sometimes alcohol can enhance or magnify the effects of medications with hazardous consequences. Sleep medications and alcohol are a particular hazard. Drinking may also cause you to forget to take medication, or to forget that you already took your medication, so that you end up taking more.

Anyone with a specific medical condition that would be aggravated by the consumption of alcohol should also abstain. Certainly those with a history of alcohol abuse fall into this category, but often people with high blood pressure, liver disease, and lots of other medical conditions should avoid alcohol. Always check with your doctor.

## THE BARE ESSENTIALS

How many calories do I need for the day to hold my weight? How many calories to lose weight?

Find yourself in the table below. It tells you how many calories you need to maintain weight, depending on your activity level. To figure out whether you're "sedentary," "moderately active," or "very active," here are the official definitions:

- **Sedentary**: The light physical activity associated with day-to-day life. Translation: This is the average person. Busy? Yes, but sedentary. (Sedentary doesn't mean bedridden.)
- **Moderately active**: Walking about 1½ to 3 miles per day at a brisk pace (like you *have* to get where you're going) or the equivalent. This would be about 30–60 minutes daily.
- **Active**: Walking more than 3 miles per day at a brisk pace, or the equivalent. This would be about 60 minutes or more of physical activity daily.

| Gender | Age (years) | Sedentary | Moderate activity | Active |
|--------|-------------|-----------|-------------------|--------|
| Child | 2–3 | 1,000 | 1,000–1,400 | 1,000–1,400 |
| Female | 4–8 | 1,200 | 1,400–1,600 | 1,400–1,800 |
|  | 9–13 | 1,600 | 1,600–2,000 | 1,800–2,200 |
|  | 14–18 | 1,800 | 2,000 | 2,400 |
|  | 19–30 | 2,000 | 2,000–2,200 | 2,400 |
|  | 31–50 | 1,800 | 2,000 | 2,200 |
|  | 51+ | 1,600 | 1,800 | 2,000–2,200 |
| Male | 4–8 | 1,400 | 1,400–1,600 | 1,600–2,000 |
|  | 9–13 | 1,800 | 1,800–2,200 | 2,000–2,600 |
|  | 14–18 | 2,200 | 2,400–2,600 | 2,800–3,200 |
|  | 19–30 | 2,400 | 2,600–2,800 | 3,000 |
|  | 31–50 | 2,200 | 2,400–2,600 | 2,800–3,000 |
|  | 51+ | 2,000 | 2,200–2,400 | 2,400–2,800 |

Note: These calorie levels are estimates and are for weight maintenance. These values assume that your weight is what it should be. For weight loss, you need to create a deficit of calories (eat less than what you need). To do this, you have some choices:

- eat fewer calories
- be more active
- a little of both

Doing a little of both allows you to still eat a fair amount because you're raising your needs with the extra activity. Also, most of us need a little more activity anyway, so it's a good fit.

To lose about a pound of fat per week, aim for a deficit of about 500 calories per day. This level is safe for most people, and it's fast enough without driving you crazy. I certainly wouldn't want obese kids losing faster than this. Indeed, I'm thrilled with this level of weight loss in obese kids. At this rate, you're down 52 pounds per year (if you even have to lose that much)! Besides, the goal here is a better lifestyle—with food and activity. Weight normalization comes second. Remember, slow and steady will win the race.

## Uncle Sam's "gotta-haves"

Here are the foods you want to include every day and the approximate amounts of each. Let's look at what we really need in our diets for good health and just how many calories it *isn't*.

| Food Category | Amount | Average calories (approx. range) |
|---|---|---|
| Fruits | 2 cups | 240 (100–300) |
| Vegetables | 2½ cups | 125 (60–400) |
| Lean meat, beans, nuts | 6 ounces | 300 (200–510) |
| Grains | 6 ounces/equivalent (3 ounces whole, 3 ounces other | 420 (420–660) |
| Low-fat/nonfat dairy | 3 cups/equivalent | 300 (240–410) |
| Fats/oils | 6 teaspoons | 200 (160–215) |
|  | **Total Basic Calories** | 1,585 (1,180–2,495) |

The ranges are approximations, because not all foods in each group have the same number of calories. Three ounces of broiled shrimp, for instance, have fewer calories than 3 ounces of salmon, but both can be included over the course of a few weeks. Likewise, apples, bananas, and pears have a few more calories than melon and berries. Vegetables can get high if you choose exclusively root vegetables like white and sweet potatoes. By all means you want some potatoes, but as part of a variety of veggies.

We don't want anyone spending time in the low end of these totals. Get 1,200 calories daily, at the very least. We recommend that, for weight loss, you focus on getting about 1,500–1,600 calories daily, and for maintenance, start with about 2,000 calories daily. Men will likely need more for maintenance and women of slight builds may need only about 1,800 calories. Of course, if you're really active, you can sock away a few hundred more calories and be none the worse for it.

## "Do-as-you-please" calories

This is the fluff. These are from whatever foods you want and no apologies needed. This is your dietary mad money. Like chocolate milk, a little full-fat cheese, a cookie or two, or a scoop of ice cream. As I've said before, I could never give up chocolate, and you shouldn't have to surrender your passions, either. The dietary guidelines actually have a sliding scale for these calories, and they get very specific, down to the exact number. We can't get that obsessive, so we just round it out.

| Total daily calories | "Do-as-you-please" calories |
| --- | --- |
| 1,500 | 150–180 |
| 1,800 | 180–200 |
| 2,000 | 200–250 |
| 2,500 | 250–400 |
| 3,000 | 300–500 |

Figure about 10 percent of your calories as "discretionary" and you'll be fine. If you need more calories overall, then you can fit in a few more of these.

## FOOD SAFETY

Food safety would never be an issue in your kitchen, right? Unsanitary kitchens are found only in those dive-type restaurants on the other side of the tracks, right? Wrong.

Fact: Most household kitchens would not pass a city health department inspection.

Sad but true, and it costs us all a lot. Did you know that each year, tens of millions of people are sickened, more than 325,000 people are hospitalized, and 5,000 people die from food poisoning? Even if it isn't fatal, it can sure ruin a nice day, or two or three, and if your mother-in-law gets it from your Thanksgiving dinner, you're toast.

Think you've never had food poisoning? Ever had the stomach flu? That was most likely food poisoning. It's true, because the classic flu symptoms do not include vomiting, cramping, and diarrhea, and food poisoning usually includes at least one of these symptoms, along with the feeling that you never want to see food again. Of course, you may not have actually eaten bad food, but there are lots of ways to get food poisoning even without wolfing down that science experiment in the back of the fridge.

Visualize this scenario: You've been cutting up chicken into parts. Your daughter asks for a glass of water and you rinse your hands and hand her a glass of water. She gets sick. She didn't really eat bad food, but her glass was contaminated with bacteria from the raw chicken. What went wrong there? You rinsed your hands but did not wash them thoroughly enough to clean them.

**Isn't food safety more of an issue for manufacturers and restaurant chains?**

That's what seems to get into the news, but most food poisoning happens in the home. Truth is, it's *everyone*'s responsibility. Food can become unsafe anytime right up to the minute you put it into your mouth, so we in the home have a lot of say-so in how safe our food is. The manufacturers and restaurants have a big stake in keeping food safe, to be sure. There's no worse publicity than the kind that comes from the news tracing the sickness of hundreds of people back to the food you sold them, so they really need to pay attention to food safety, and for the most part, they really do their jobs. All their hard work, however, can be totally undone by how we handle the food at home.

The Uncle Sam eating style works, but only when your food is handled well. Food poisoning is not a good way to lose weight. Let's look at the guidelines on food safety.

Guideline: *Clean hands, food contact surfaces, and fruits and vegetables. Meat and poultry should not be washed or rinsed.*

Let's look at each of these separately:

- Clean hands: Big point here, because 50 percent of all foodborne illness could be prevented by good hand washing. That means soap and water, vigorous washing for 20 seconds, and thorough rinsing. (How long is 20 seconds? Longer than you think. Hum or sing "Happy Birthday" twice while you wash your hands. The song takes about 20 seconds.)
- Food contact surfaces: Make sure whatever you put the food on is clean. Knives and food prep utensils need to be clean, too.
- Fruits and vegetables: Wash them! Even if they're organic, you can't tell if they rolled off

the truck and onto a road traveled by farm animals (get the picture?). Be sure to wash even fruits and veggies where you don't eat the outside. If there is crud on the rind of a melon, the knife pushes the crud inside when you slice. As for ready-to-eat packaged salads, they're okay to eat as is, but only if they've been kept refrigerated and eaten by the use-by date.

- Meat, poultry, and fish: Rinsing is just a huge opportunity to spread surface bacteria and is really unnecessary. Think of all the splattering that goes on when you rinse. Our view: If the meat/poultry/fish needs rinsing to be edible, you probably shouldn't eat it anyway. Enough said.

Guideline: *Separate raw, cooked, and ready-to-eat foods while shopping, preparing, and storing foods.*

The idea here is that you don't put the packages of raw meat in the same bag as the fresh bread, fruits, and veggies. The juices from the raw meat can drip onto the produce and contaminate it. And you might never know until you, or someone in the household, get sick.

One common scene: Guys always want to do the grilling of the meat. Somehow they think they came out of the womb knowing all about grilling. Okay, fine, but they don't necessarily know about how to keep that grilled meat and chicken safe and clean. Often they take the marinated raw meat out of the dish, grill it and put it right back into the dish it was marinated in, "so you don't waste any of the marinade." You also don't waste the bacteria that were on the raw meat/chicken and put that right back on the clean, finished product. Keep raw meat *and any surfaces it touched* separate from the cooked product and anything else that is ready to eat.

---

BUY PLASTIC CUTTING BOARDS IN DIFFERENT COLORS. USE THE RED BOARD ONLY FOR MEAT, POULTRY, AND FISH. GREEN IS FOR FRUIT AND VEGETABLES. YELLOW IS FOR EVERYTHING ELSE—CHEESE, BREAD, ETC. THEY ARE DISHWASHER SAFE, BUT THAT MAY NOT KILL EVERY SINGLE GERM. SEPARATE, DON'T CROSS-CONTAMINATE.

SOME PEOPLE WIPE UP THE RAW CHICKEN JUICE FROM THE COUNTER, AND THEN USE THAT SAME SPONGE TO WASH THE DISHES (YOU KNOW WHO YOU ARE). THIS IS A RECIPE FOR DISASTER. WIPE UP SPILLS WITH PAPER TOWELS. TO DISINFECT YOUR SPONGE, ZAP IT IN THE MICROWAVE OR PUT IT IN THE DISHWASHER. DO THIS *OFTEN*.

---

Guideline: *Cook foods to a safe temperature to kill microorganisms.*

Even if you memorize the diagram below, you'll never know for sure if your food reaches a safe temperature *unless you test it with a meat thermometer.* A meat thermometer is the most important utensil in your kitchen! It's also one of the cheapest. You can pick up a very decent one for about $10. That's way cheaper than a visit to the doctor. Taking the temperature of your food is also way easier than taking a child's temperature, too, because the food never moves around.

Bacteria really have a party between the temperatures of 40° and 140° Farhenheit. That's when they breed like rabbits. Above that temperature, some foods need to be cooked to higher temperatures than others, as you can see.

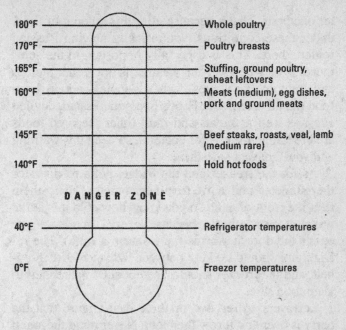

| | |
|---|---|
| 180°F | Whole poultry |
| 170°F | Poultry breasts |
| 165°F | Stuffing, ground poultry, reheat leftovers |
| 160°F | Meats (medium), egg dishes, pork and ground meats |
| 145°F | Beef steaks, roasts, veal, lamb (medium rare) |
| 140°F | Hold hot foods |

**DANGER ZONE**

| | |
|---|---|
| 40°F | Refrigerator temperatures |
| 0°F | Freezer temperatures |

Source: 2005 U.S. Dietary Guidelines for Americans

---

**Cooking school 101:** The benefit of taking the temperature of meat/poultry:

- You'll finally know when it's done!
- No more overcooked meat!
- You get hamburgers instead of hockey pucks and turkey that is so moist it doesn't need gravy!

---

Guideline: *Chill (refrigerate) perishable foods promptly and defrost foods properly.*

The "food safety" definition of "promptly" is this: Refrigerate leftovers after two hours. When the temperature is 80° Fahrenheit or above, then refrigerate after one hour. That's because after this amount of time, under these conditions, you're really playing Russian roulette here. This is especially important in the summertime or whenever the weather is hot (think picnics and outdoor barbecues), when people want to keep food out all afternoon. Foods like potato salad, deviled eggs, as well as meats and most other prepared foods are breeding grounds for bacteria, so heed this warning and you'll have a safe meal.

As for the freezer and the fridge, get a refrigerator thermometer and a freezer thermometer. Hang them near the front of each so you know how cold it is at the warmest part (that's because every time someone opens the door it warms the front up a little). The refrigerator should be kept between 32° and 40° Fahrenheit, and the freezer should be kept at 0° Fahrenheit to keep food safe.

Leftovers: After two or three days, figure that the party is over and throw them out. Never mind the smell test here—it doesn't tell you the truth. Food goes bad before it smells bad. Wrap leftovers in small containers so they'll chill quickly. The cliché holds: When in doubt, throw it out.

Guideline: *Avoid raw (unpasteurized) milk and any products made from unpasteurized milk, raw or partially cooked eggs, or any foods containing raw eggs, raw or undercooked meat, raw or undercooked meat or poultry, unpasteurized juices and raw sprouts.*

**The boil-down**: We've all had situations where we, or those we know, have eaten some or all of these foods and had no problems. Dr. Keith even grew up in

California—the land of the alfalfa sprout—and he's had his share of those avocado sandwiches with sprouts, yada, yada, yada. But he doesn't eat them now because raw sprouts can harbor some bad microorganisms. Doesn't mean *all* sprouts have them, but again, it's the Russian roulette thing. If you lose, you really pay big. Five thousand people each year die from foodborne sickness. It's just not worth the risk. The same goes for raw milk and unpasteurized juice.

All of the above can seem scary, but it's really not. We don't want you to feel that you have to prepare for surgery before fixing dinner. No need for latex here, just some common sense and lots of hand washing, before and after preparing food, and also during, whenever you change tasks.

There's lots of good info on food safety at these Web sites:

- www.homefoodsafety.org
- www.foodsafety.gov
- www.fightbac.org

## PACKING A POWER PANTRY

It's get-real time. If you want to make an omelet, you have to break a few eggs. But first you need the eggs—and everything else that goes with them. Keep the following on hand and you'll have what you need to eat well:

## Foods

- Olive oil and a neutral oil, like canola. Use olive oil for flavor; canola for baking.
- Cooking spray, especially the butter-flavored one for popcorn. Spray veggies before grilling so you can coat but not drench with oil.
- Balsamic vinegar is worth the investment. It adds taste, but not fat, to salads and grilled vegetables.
- Trans-free tub margarine (like Smart Balance or Promise Spread)—the benefits of margarine without the trans fat. Of course, a little butter is nice sometimes, too.
- Eggs. Incredible nutrition, edible at any meal, and the original fast food.
- Onions and garlic. What would Italy, Spain, France, or any enlightened cook do without them?
- Canned tomato paste, tomatoes, and sauce. Try to find the ones with no added salt, but don't go crazy. They're good either way.
- Canned beans—kidney, garbanzo, black, pink, and any others you like. They're cheap and hearty and you can sneak them in anywhere for added protein and fiber.
- Pasta, including the pasta "blends" with whole wheat added. Great vehicles for veggies and beans, fish, and any sauce under the sun.
- Whole-grain cereals (Cheerios, Raisin bran, whole wheat flakes, etc.).
- Oatmeal: quick-cooking, unsweetened and individual ready sweetened. No time to cook it? Just add cold milk and eat.

- Bulgur. Just soak it and it's ready for tabbouleh, and cooked it's great for pilaf.
- Whole wheat and white flour. Mix them together for most of your baking.
- Brown and white rice, because white has lots of folic acid and iron.
- Nuts, especially almonds and walnuts, with heart healthy omega-3 fat.
- Peanut butter. It's comfort with nutrition.
- Milk powder (you'll find it near the cocoa mixes). Throw it in pancake mix, your coffee, a smoothie. Great protein/calcium booster.
- Cocoa powder. Way better for hot chocolate than the envelopes!
- Spices: garlic powder, pepper, chili powder, cumin, Italian herbs, oregano, thyme, yada, yada—use as desired and experiment. No calories!
- Mustard (yellow or go for the fancy whole grain type)—actually has some antioxidants and no calories, so pour it on.
- Light yogurt, flavored and unflavored—all the nutrition of a glass of milk.
- Sugar and other sweetener, if desired—good taste tools when you used wisely
- Frozen vegetables, especially peas and corn. They offer the same nutrition as fresh—just defrost them.

Cooking equipment/utensils

- Steamer basket—cheap and an absolute necessity
- Dutch oven—Tons of uses and it goes in the oven, too

- Wok—stir-fries those meals with lots less oil
- Tongs—like using your fingers, but without the burn
- 1-inch paintbrush (better than a pastry brush)
- Assorted spoons, metal and wooden
- Large and small skillet
- Large and small saucepan
- Ziploc bags for coating food with oil and seasonings
- Can opener (manual is fine)
- 3-sided (or 4-sided) grater
- Blender
- Hand mixer

Optional but nice

- Hot-air popper
- Food processor. I like chopping by hand, but these are good for big production work, like parties.
- Spice or coffee grinder—amazing for blending herbs and spices

# CHAPTER 4

# Uncle Sam Says You've Got to Move It to Lose It

## PHYSICAL ACTIVITY

**What's physical activity doing as part of the "Dietary" Guidelines? We know it's good to exercise, but isn't this supposed to be about food?**

Actually, the Uncle Sam Diet is about good food, good eating, and healthy living. Notice that we said "physical activity," not "exercise."

**What's the difference?**

Exercise means rules and regulations, and it conjures up nasty images of some drill sergeant barking orders to drop and give him fifty. Mention exercise to most people, especially people watching their weight, and you'll elicit moans and groans. You'll also meet a wall of resistance.

I built many of those walls myself as I was growing up. I was really lousy at most sports. Last one picked on the team, groans from teammates when I got up to bat, the works. If the sport involved throwing, catching, or any contact with a ball, fuhgeddaboutit. That eliminated football, baseball, basketball, even volleyball, although I was okay at that until I had to serve. Let's not even mention tennis. Too bad, because I had a great-uncle who, many decades ago, was involved in the formation of the California Tennis Association. Sorry, Uncle Harry. If it just didn't involve a ball . . .

Here's what Uncle Sam has to say about physical activity:

Guideline: *Engage in regular physical activity and reduce sedentary activities to promote health, psychological well-being, and a healthy body weight.*

Translation: This is a more general guideline, and the most interesting piece is the part about being active to promote "psychological well-being." Moderate physical activity does make you feel better—physically and emotionally. You may have heard of those little compounds called endorphins. Your brain makes them as a result of physical activity. They're responsible for the phenomenon called the runner's high. Don't worry, they don't get you spacey or anything; endorphins just give you a little lift, a mild feeling of euphoria. Being physically active daily can even help prevent or manage depression. It's often part of the treatment plan for people with depression.

Guideline: *Achieve physical fitness by including cardiovascular conditioning, stretching exercise for flexibility, and resistance exercises or calisthenics for muscle strength and endurance.*

Translation: Notice here that a good mix of activities is mentioned. You need to do more than one type of activity to get and stay healthy, but that's also the fun of it. Some days you just don't feel like doing this or that, but you can do something else. You can also mix things up on any particular day. Yard work can be a bit of both cardiovascular and resistance activities, especially if you're in the yard for a while and doing some serious planting, mowing, and lifting all those bags of soil. Stretching, for example, is good after activity and to warm up before. It also can help release a lot of tension.

**Cardiovascular and resistance activity—what are the differences?**

Physical activity can be broken down into two basic types:

- resistance (aka anaerobic or strength training)
- cardiovascular (aka aerobic)

They're both important, but they do different things. Resistance activities are very intense ones that you do for a short time. Weight lifting is an example. Bench pressing for ten reps, arm curls with barbells, like that. Chin-ups and sit-ups (crunches) are also resistance activities. They build strength and muscle. More muscle means you can eat more calories because it takes calories to keep muscles fed and happy. That's why pro athletes, especially very muscular ones, can eat huge portions of food. It's also why men have an easier time losing weight. Take a man and a woman, each 5'7" and

150 pounds. The man needs more calories each day because he will almost always have more muscle. It's genetic. Don't shoot the messenger; I didn't decide any of this.

Cardiovascular activities strengthen your heart. The heart is a muscle, but it doesn't need to be bigger, just stronger. Think swimming, dancing, bicycling, tennis, rowing, stair climbing, and just plain walking. Walking is one of the best aerobic activities, in fact. Your heart gets stronger by doing activities for longer periods of time but at a lower intensity.

**How much of this "physical activity" do we need each day?**

Well, let's look at the guidelines, which spell it out. Then we'll talk about them afterward.

> Guideline: *To reduce the risk of chronic disease in adulthood: Engage in at least 30 minutes of moderate-intensity physical activity, above usual activity, at work or home on most days of the week.*

Translation: This is for most people who are already within a normal weight range. Note two things here: "moderate-intensity" activity and "above usual activity."

Check the table below for examples of moderate- and vigorous-intensity activity. "Above usual activity" means that you won't get away with saying, "Oh I'm already active at the office."

| Moderate physical activity | Approximate calories burned per hour for a 154-pound person |
|---|---|
| Hiking | 370 |
| Light gardening/yard work | 330 |
| Dancing | 330 |
| Golf (walking and carrying clubs) | 330 |
| Bicycling (<10 mph) | 290 |
| Walking (3½ mph) | 280 |
| Weight lifting (general light workout) | 220 |
| Stretching | 180 |
| **Vigorous physical activity** | |
| Running/jogging (5 mph) | 590 |
| Bicycling (>10 mph) | 590 |
| Swimming (slow, freestyle laps) | 510 |
| Aerobics | 480 |
| Walking ( 4½ mph) | 460 |
| Heavy yard work (like chopping wood) | 440 |
| Weight lifting (vigorous effort) | 440 |
| Basketball (vigorous) | 440 |

Note to self: Busy doesn't mean Active.

You say you're very busy, and I absolutely believe that you are. But that's not the same as being active. You can be busy constantly at work without ever leaving your desk, and always get exhausted by the end of the day. You're still not active. Ironically, becoming more physically active might actually make it easier to get through the day, and it can even give you more energy and put you into a better mood.

Guideline: *To help manage body weight and prevent gradual, unhealthy weight gain in adulthood: Engage in approximately 60 minutes of moderate- to vigorous-intensity physical activity on most days of the week while not exceeding caloric intake requirements.*

**The boil-down**: If you want to keep the weight off as you get older, you may need to do more than 30 minutes on most days. It may take up to 60 minutes. This is assuming that you don't overdo the calories, too. You may be able to eat a few more without gaining weight. Just keep a level head about it, because your waistline has an incredible accounting system.

Guideline: *To sustain weight loss in adulthood: Participate in at least 60 to 90 minutes of daily moderate-intensity physical activity while not exceeding caloric intake requirements. Some people may need to consult a healthcare provider before participating in this level of activity.*

**The boil-down**: Take a deep breath and relax. No need to panic. You don't have to spend 90 minutes every day on a treadmill in order to be healthy into adulthood. Here's the deal: You've lost some weight and you want to keep it off. You can absolutely do it, and being active makes it easier. In fact, being active is what makes it possible.

**The statistics on regaining lost weight are horrible. Can anyone realistically lose weight and keep it off?**

Absolutely! We in the research world seem to study only what fails and then we try to figure out why. Let's switch gears and study the successes. That's what Dr. James Hill of the University of Colorado and Dr. Regina Wing of Brown University and the University of Pittsburgh did when they started the National Weight Control Registry. They compiled thousands of people who had objective proof that they had lost at least 30 pounds and kept it off for at least a year. You can check it out for yourself at www.nwcr.ws. Then he and his team asked this question: What did successful weight maintainers have in common?

Several things, but not how they lost their weight. Some did it on their own, some joined group programs like Weight Watchers, others did liquid diets or low-carb diets or other fad diets. So they lost weight in different ways, but they *kept it off* in very similar ways. Here's how most did it:

- A balanced, generally low-fat diet. (It was about 24 percent of calories from fat, but people often underreport their fat intake, so figure closer to 30 percent)
- A positive attitude, with many sources of pleasure and happiness in life, not only food.
- Physical activity! Most did about 60 minutes for at least 5 days per week. Walking was the most common activity.

That's from the successful cases, and I'm not going to argue with them. Think of what the successful people had in common:

- They were motivated and determined, and they stayed that way.
- They called it a day with their old eating habits and changed them.
- They also kept food in perspective and realized that it's important, but so are other pleasures.
- They learned to really enjoy their activity.

So how do you start enjoying physical activity?

First, make the payoff more than just managing or losing weight. The payoff has to be even more than better health. That's good for some people, but diehard haters of anything physical need more. For them the payoff from doing physical activity might be that it helps them to calm down and slow up a bit, and gives them another way to unplug, maybe even have some fun.

Physical activity doesn't have to crowd out your fun. For the successful weight maintainers, it became a part of their enjoyment. Make it a part of your fun as well. Physical activities that are social can help do this. For some that means a team sports. Others may want something where they can feel like a kid again. You wouldn't believe what happens when couples take up some kind of dancing—ballroom dancing, square dancing, Scottish country dancing, even tap (I'm talking of people you'd never expect to like dancing). It's a way to let off some steam and be social. I also had a patient who grew to like doing charity walkathons. She would get together with a few friends and do a 5-, a 10-, or even an 18-mile walkathon. She said they would just have a long conversation while they were walking, instead of sitting around on the phone with each other or hanging out.

Little hint for happy living: *Any* new activity feels awkward at first. For crying out loud, so did taking your first steps when you were a baby, but you stayed with it, right? Good. Now, repeat that principle. Persistence pays off.

My suggestions when thinking of becoming more physically active:

- Resolve that you need to do *something*.
- Choose something you like, or that you'd like to try. If you've always hated physical activity, you may need to choose something that you "dislike the least."
- Think of ways to make your activity more enjoyable and motivating. Get creative here. If wearing a hot pink tutu while you go walking gets you charged up about walking, do it. Anything goes, if it works for you.
- Go slow. Like with changing your eating style, I don't care how fast you change. Think about where you want to be next year at this time, not next week.
- Make it a priority. It's that important. *You're* that important. The world can spin without you for 30 minutes.

- Keep track of your progress! It's very motivating to know roughly how many calories you've burned or how far you walked, ran, or swam.

**A word about walking**: It's the least expensive and most available activity, and it has real physical and emotional benefits. It's also the easiest activity to start and you can feel like a pro from day 1. The America on the Move program is a great example. It promotes getting people to increase their level of physical activity, especially in easy, simple ways like just by walking more. Dr. Jim Hill was among those who got this ball rolling, and it's taken off around the country. Bravo again, Dr. Hill and gang. Learn more at www.america onthemove.org.

### How to walk smart

- Get a pedometer. You can buy one for less than $10. Hook it on to your belt and keep it with you for a few days so you can get an average step count for a day.
- Aim to get 2,000 steps per day *more* than you usually get. That's only about a mile.
- Increase at your own pace and one that you can maintain on most days.
- A good goal is to get to 10,000 steps per day, or about five miles. (Okay, five miles is a lot—but it includes all those steps to and from the fridge.)
- Keep a record of your progress. It's a good math project for the kids.

The point is to make little changes at a time. To change permanently, you need to change gradually. So let go of the time factor and trade it for consistency. It'll get you way farther and do it better. Get pedometers for your entire family. Give them as gifts. Kids especially love to track their progress. For more hints, check out the Web site at www.americaonthemove.org.

**Do I have to join a gym?**

No. You can walk or jog for free—that's one reason there are sidewalks.

But a gym has many pluses. There are lots of exercise classes, which make working out social—and remember, misery loves company (though after a while it becomes fun). Don't worry if you are a klutz. There is always someone else who is just as clumsy. And this isn't school; you don't get graded. Also, you'll improve.

There is lots of equipment, from aerobic machines like bikes and treadmills and StairMasters to resistance machines for every part of the body, including muscles you didn't know existed.

There is staff to help you.

There usually are perks—Jacuzzi, steam room, sauna.

Three things to consider:

- Is the gym convenient to your home or office? If it is more than a few blocks away, you have too many excuses not to go: it's too hot out, too cold, too rainy.
- There is no point joining a gym if you won't actually go. Most gyms offer a brief (and cheap)

trial membership so you can see if a gym is for you without committing to a whole year.

- Check out what people are wearing. If the leotard matches the tights, which match the leg warmers, which match the sneakers, it's intimidating (and, to my mind, overachieving). You want a workout arena, not a fashion show. Look for a gym where the best-dressed person is just someone whose T-shirt isn't torn.

## Do I need a trainer?

Sure, if money is no object. Trainers are expensive ($100 an hour in one big New York City chain of health clubs).

If you are using the machines and/or free weights, you do need a couple of sessions with a trainer—on your first day, a week later, maybe two weeks after that. You need to learn how to use the apparatus correctly, and how to use it for *you*. You have a bad back? Your knees aren't what they used to be? You couldn't touch your toes if someone offered you $1 million? There's a weird pain in your shoulder? You need some guidance and supervision.

A trainer will work out an exercise plan for you. He or she will keep you on track and make sure that you are progressing. He or she should revise your plan every so often so you don't get bored. He or she will praise you for your good efforts.

Consider having a session with a trainer at least once a month. You've already eliminated a drink or two after work with your friends—in a month, that probably comes to $100.

## When is the best time to do physical activity?

Whenever you *will* do it. Some like the early morning, some like after work. Others do it on their lunch hour. Whatever floats your boat is fine here. Sometimes you need to be a little flexible. Maybe you planned to go for a walk on your lunch hour but work got nuts. No problem, just go later in the day or after work. Indeed, some moderate activity after work is a great stress buster. It may help keep you from needing that drink to unwind.

**Little hint for happy living**: Doing vigorous exercise right before bedtime might keep you awake a little longer, so finish your physical activity a couple of hours before you go to bed if you have difficulty sleeping.

### Here are some other ways to step lively

- Turn errands into activity time. Go for a brisk walk to the greengrocer or supermarket for today's salad greens or even a quart of milk.
- Stop delivery of the Sunday paper so you'll have to walk to the store to get it. (One of my things to do. I *really* want my Sunday paper, so it gets me up and out the door and walking a mile each way. If I do nothing else that day, I've at least walked for a couple of miles.)
- Turn the family pet into an opportunity for daily activity. Fido will appreciate more than just a backyard break. He needs to go on different walks and he'd happily let you come along. Pets need physical activity too. Ask your vet: Pets are getting fatter, too. We're giving them our

sedentary ways and too-large portions and it's giving them health problems!

- Take walks after dinner. Bring a friend. Bring your kids.
- Turn your lunch hour into a half hour of lunch and a half hour of walking. It won't get you too sweaty for the office and it knocks off a good chunk of your activity gig for the day. Walk first, then pick up lunch on the way back.
- Keep it exciting. Vary your activities with the seasons, so you can be active all year long. Hike in the fall, ski in the winter, you know the drill. If you're lucky enough to join a gym with a pool, you can swim all year, or take a water aerobics classes.

# CHAPTER 5

# Guidelines for Special Situations and Special Groups with Special Needs

## DINING OUT

At home, controlling what you eat is easier. What happens when life intervenes and takes us on the road—either at work, for the evening, or on a trip?

You wouldn't go on any trip without planning, and eating out requires a plan. Face it, when it comes to eating well, restaurants do not always have your health at heart. Their number one concern is how the food tastes, not what it will do to your waistline or blood pressure. Little wonder that restaurant meals are often high in fat, salt, and sugar. Portions are often large, huge, or gargantuan. Understand this and you'll be able to work around it all and still have a great time eating out.

Most people's eating styles could be called spontaneous, at best. They fly by the seat of their pants, eat impulsively and compulsively, whatever is within reach when they're hungry, and eventually the seat of their pants gets so large that they can't get off the ground.

Ya gotta have a plan. Call it a "food policy." Most of us know when we'll be eating out socially. To make sure you'll be as happy at the end of the meal as you were when you started, here are some strategies:

- Eat lighter on dining-out days. Keep the other two meals lean, with lots of high-volume fruit and veggies to chomp on during the day to keep filled.
- Definitely get some physical activity:
  - Walk to the restaurant.
  - Go for a brisk walk on your lunch hour.
  - Hit the gym early.
  - Walk home afterward.
- **E.A.T.:** a great 150-calorie premeal snack to prevent overeating at a party or a restaurant:
  - **E**gg (hard-cooked)
  - **A**pple
  - **T**hirst quencher (water, seltzer, or calorie-free beverage)
- **C.A.T.:** Same as above, but substitute an ounce of cheese for the egg. It will curb your hunger and let you focus on the event, not just the food.
- Scope out restaurant menus for low-calorie options. Grilled, broiled, poached, seared, boiled, baked, and steamed foods have less fat and fewer calories than fried or sautéed anything.
- Order once, eat twice: Resolve to take half of the meal home for the next day. If you like the meal, it's a great reprise. If you don't, you haven't eaten calories you didn't really want.
- Order a salad, then get another appetizer as your entrée. Often appetizers are the best part of the

menu. Ask for dressings on the side, so you'll dip, not drown in, added fat and calories.

- Soup's on! Go for broth-based or tomato-based soups like chicken noodle and minestrone, or consommé and save the cream-based ones for when you get a taste of someone else's.
- Choose tomato-based sauces instead of white or cream-based sauces on meat, fish, and pasta.
- Order carefully if you know you want dessert. And if you do, share it. Or make dessert a cappuccino with whole milk. Have it with real sugar and it's still only about 150 calories and luscious. It even counts toward your milk for the day.

## GOING THE DISTANCE

For many people, traveling means hitting one rest stop after another, and fries come with that. You can do better, and really easily:

- Travel with sturdy fresh fruit and veggies. Oranges, pears, and apples are great for long trips.
- Grab a low-fat ice cream or frozen yogurt cone to keep hunger at bay during a layover.
- Go nuts at the airport! Bring along packs of dried fruit and nuts to nibble a little at a time during those endless waits.
- Cinnamon gum keeps its flavor longer and your taste buds stimulated.
- Water, water, water . . . especially in planes, where humidity is so low.

- Airport snack bars now have lots of options packed to go: yogurt, fruit salad, small packs of nuts, low-fat wraps, even fat-free muffins.
- Don't give up on fast food, but have it your way. Choose salad, baked potatoes, low-fat milk, juice and water, even fresh fruit and low-fat ice cream. Craving fries and a burger? Order the smallest size of each and add a green salad.
- Dashboard dining? The best one-handed, no-mess fruits are strawberries, apples, and pears. Diced low-fat cheese, nuts (fill that empty Altoids or Velamints tin and they'll stay put), soy nuts, and whole wheat pretzels all make good traveling companions.

## SPECIAL GROUPS WITH SPECIAL NEEDS

### Adults over fifty

Guideline: *People over age 50: Get your vitamin B$_{12}$ from fortified foods or supplements.*

Translation: As we get older, we have a harder time absorbing natural vitamin B$_{12}$ from food. B$_{12}$ is naturally found in all animal foods, but the synthetic form is in fortified cereals and of course in multivitamin supplements. This is one of the times when synthetic is a little better than natural, because we can absorb B$_{12}$ more easily in the synthetic form. No problem. Take a multivitamin daily (menopausal women: get vitamin without iron), or have fortified whole grain cereal on most days and consider the problem solved.

Guideline: *Older Adults: Participate in regular physical activity to reduce functional declines associated with aging and to achieve the other benefits of physical activity identified for all adults.*

The bottom line here is that muscles stay around only if there's a demand for them. It's use 'em or lose 'em. Physical activity also helps preserve good coordination skills and mental alertness. Besides, when you're older you actually *do* have more time! But older people also have to respect their bodies and ease into activity gradually. It's not about being a hero, just being more active more often.

Guideline: *Older adults: Only eat certain deli meats and frankfurters that have been reheated to steaming hot.*

Most deli meats and frankfurters are fine most of the time. But some deli meats, especially cured meats and frankfurters, have been associated with outbreaks of a sometimes fatal foodborne illness caused by an organism called *listeria monocytogenes,* commonly known just as listeria. You can still eat these foods *if they are heated to steaming hot.* Our suggestion is, if you really want a frankfurter or deli meat, prepare it yourself so it's steaming hot. That way you know for sure how it was cooked and handled.

Guideline: *Older adults: Do not eat or drink raw (unpasteurized) milk or any products made from unpasteurized milk, raw or undercooked eggs, or any foods containing raw eggs, raw or undercooked meat or poultry, unpasteurized juices and raw sprouts, raw or undercooked fish or shellfish.*

This is basically the same food guideline given earlier, with one exception: no raw fish or shellfish for this group. You don't have the same defenses as the rest of us and it's harder for you to kill or fight bacteria you ingest. So hold the sushi, please, and stay away from any oyster that isn't cooked. Incidentally, although cooked fish is fine for these groups, some restaurants get snooty and ask things like, "How would you like your salmon cooked, Madame? Rare is how the chef suggests." Rare means that it's undercooked. Tell him or her that Monsieur or Madame would like the salmon cooked through, please. The same holds true for beef and lamb. At least go for medium. It might not be rare, but it's not as risky, either, especially since you can't be there to take its temperature, and medium should put you in the safe zone.

Guideline: *Older adults and people exposed to insufficient ultraviolet-band radiation (i.e. sunlight): Consume extra vitamin D from vitamin D–fortified foods and/or sunlight.*

No need to bake in the sun to get your vitamin D. But many older people, can't make vitamin D as easily. Also, if you live in a cold climate where you have to stay covered up and indoors for the winter, or if you wear sunscreen regularly, you may not get enough sunshine to make enough vitamin D. That's yet another reason to drink milk, mostly low-fat and fat-free milk.

It's the best dietary source of vitamin D we have. Next best are multivitamin supplements with vitamin D. This vitamin is a major player in helping you to use the calcium you're getting, so help yourself out and drink your three-a-day of dairy foods.

Guideline: *Special guidelines for special people: Older adults: aim to get no more than 1,500 mg. of sodium per day, and meet the potassium recommendation (4,700 mg./day) with food.*

As we get older, we tend to get more sensitive to the effects of salt. Check with your physician at your next physical. If you don't have high blood pressure, then aim for 2,300 milligrams of sodium per day and be glad you're healthy.

· This isn't rocket science. You'll bring your salt intake down just by subbing some fresh fruits for the usual salty snacks. The bottom line is that this is yet another reason to eat your fruits and veggies. Simple stuff like this, along with keeping active, can really lower your blood pressure. Just think of the perks:

• feeling better
• doing more with daily life
• less chance of a stroke or a heart attack
• fewer medications with side effects like sexual dysfunction and lots more

Note the emphasis on getting potassium *from food*, not salt substitutes, supplements, or pills. Salt substitutes are really just potassium chloride. They come in shakers, much like salt, and you can find them in the supermarket right where you get salt.

Salt substitutes don't mix with some medications, and they aren't good for people with some medical conditions, especially people who have certain types of kidney diseases. The same holds true for potassium pills or supplements. You really need clearance from your physician before you use salt substitutes or potassium supplements or pills. One other thing that may keep you from trying salt substitutes: They don't exactly taste like salt. They tend to taste metallic.

If you rely on supplements to meet your potassium needs, you probably aren't getting all the fruits and vegetables and low-fat dairy foods you need, so start right there. Food is powerful health, and it tastes way better than pills. Besides, you'll never get into a pill what you can get from a good, healthy eating style. And aren't you glad? Talk about taking the fun out of life. Personally, I'm glad they haven't figured out how to get healthy eating into a pill. I enjoy my meals too much, and I really want you to have the same pleasures from eating, too.

### Women who are pregnant or breast-feeding

Guideline: *Women of childbearing age who may become pregnant: Eat foods high in heme-iron, and/or consume iron-rich plant foods or fortified foods with an enhancer of iron absorption, such as vitamin C–rich foods.*

Heme-iron comes from animal sources like meat and fish. If you get iron from whole grains and fortified grains, beans, and dark, leafy greens, then something with vitamin C or other acid helps you absorb it better, that's all. A vinaigrette with that spinach salad is what we're talking about here. Some strawberries or a glass of orange juice with your whole-grain cereal or toast. Or just have some fruit for dessert most of the time and again, problem solved.

Guideline: *Women of childbearing age who may become pregnant and those in the first trimester of pregnancy: Consume adequate synthetic folic acid daily (from fortified foods or supplements) in addition to food forms of folate from a varied diet.*

This is the other case where synthetic nutrients are better absorbed. Most pregnant women take pregnancy multivitamins that have adequate folate. This is great for preventing some birth defects, like spina bifida, and is now in all enriched grains. Just remember to take your supplements if they're prescribed!

Guideline: *Pregnant women: Ensure proper weight gain as specified by a healthcare provider.*

The story here is that pregnancy is serious business. No, the world won't collapse if you eat a red jelly bean, but pregnancy is not a license to eat for two from day one, either. And exercise is possible and even recommended during most of your pregnancy, if your health is good. Follow you health-care provider's recommendations closely, and your pregnancy can be a great experience.

Guideline: *Breastfeeding women: Moderate weight reduction is safe and does not compromise the weight gain of the nursing infant.*

Indeed, during the average pregnancy, your body lays down an extra 7 to 10 pounds of fat in order to fuel the production of breast milk once the baby arrives. If you don't breast-feed, that fat stays there. (How many women do you know who say, "I gained about 10 pounds with each baby?"). On the other hand, gradual weight reduction during breast-feeding is not only safe, it's more or less a normal event.

Guideline: *Pregnant Women: In the absence of medical or obstetric complications, incorporate 30 minutes or more of moderate-intensity physical activity on most, if not all, days of the week. Avoid activities with a high risk of falling or abdominal trauma.*

Pregnancy is a pretty normal condition, in the absence of medical conditions, and as long as you use some common sense, you can still be active while you're pregnant. Indeed, it can provide you with the same benefits as being active does when you're not pregnant. And remember, for most of your pregnancy, you really aren't "eating for two." Stay in shape when you're pregnant and it'll be easier to get back in shape after the blessed event arrives. Of course, the accent is on common sense and check with your doctor just to get the okay for activity and for any limitations, especially if you want to do anything more than moderate-intensity activities.

Guideline: *Breastfeeding Women: Be aware that neither acute nor regular exercise adversely affects the
mother's ability to breastfeed.*

I admit it, I've never breastfed. But this guideline is
here to reassure women that physical activity is perfectly fine for you and won't reduce production of
breast milk or interfere at all. Just don't breast-feed
while you're on the treadmill.

Guideline: *Pregnant women: Only eat certain deli
meats and frankfurters that have been reheated to
steaming hot.*

Most deli meats and frankfurters are fine most of
the time. But some deli meats, especially cured
meats and frankfurters, have been associated with
outbreaks of a sometimes fatal foodborne illness
caused by an organism called *listeria monocytogenes,* commonly known just as listeria. You can still
heat these foods *if they are heated to steaming hot.*
Our suggestion is, if you really want a frankfurter or
deli meat, prepare it yourself so it's steaming hot.
That way you know for sure how it was cooked and
handled.

Guideline: *Pregnant women: Do not eat or drink raw
(unpasteurized) milk or any products made from unpasteurized milk, raw or undercooked eggs, or any
foods containing raw eggs, raw or undercooked meat
or poultry, unpasteurized juices and raw sprouts, raw
or undercooked fish or shellfish.*

This is basically the same food guideline given earlier, with one exception: no raw fish or shellfish for this group. You don't have the same defenses as the rest of us and it's harder for you to kill or fight bacteria you ingest. So hold the sushi, please, and stay away from any oyster that isn't cooked. Incidentally, although cooked fish is fine, for some restaurants get snooty and ask things like, "How would you like your salmon cooked, Madame? Rare is how the chef suggests." Rare means that it's undercooked. Tell him or her that Monsieur or Madame would like the salmon cooked through, please. The same holds true for beef and lamb. At least go for medium. It might not be rare, but it's not as risky, either, especially since you can't be there to take its temperature, and medium should put you in the safe zone.

### Children and adolescents

Guideline: *Children and Adolescents: Engage in at least 60 minutes of physical activity on most, preferably all, days of the week.*

This is a lot easier if you just cut "screen time" of all sorts (TV, video/computer games, hand-held game gizmos, the Internet, etc.) to a max of two hours daily.

Guideline: *Special grain guideline for children & adolescents: Consume whole grain foods often. At least half the grains should be whole grain.*

In short, no need to prepare foods separately for children. Take them along on the whole grain ride. Aim for three servings daily for sure.

Guideline: *Special dairy guidelines for kids: Children 2 to 8 years old should get 2 cups per day of fat-free or low-fat milk or equivalent milk products. Children 9 years of age or older should consume 3 cups per day of fat-free or low-fat milk or equivalent milk products.*

The bottom line here is that as kids grow and their calorie needs increase, so do their calcium needs. Should a two-year-old drink fat-free milk? It's fine after age two. But rather than shift all at once, think of changing over during the course of a year. If your kids prefer low-fat milk (1 percent) over fat-free, it's fine also. I want to make sure they drink milk.

Guideline: *For overweight children: Reduce the rate of weight gain while allowing growth and development. Consult a healthcare provider before placing a child on a weight-reduction diet.*

I can't say this more strongly: If your child is significantly overweight, take action—but don't do it alone because you're in over your head. Talk to your pediatrician and get the help of a registered dietitian. It'll save you a lot of time and frustration, and it'll probably be easier than you think. Kids are growing beings, so even stabilizing their weight can allow them to "grow into" their weight.

What any parent can do with a clear conscience is reduce some of the empty calories—sodas, chips, and sweets—and never use food as a reward. Believe it or not, kids do just fine with a better diet. They often like how much better they feel, too, and that helps them feel a whole lot better about themselves. They can't do this on their own, so we need to help them and get them help if we need to.

## Individuals with Medical Conditions

> Guideline: *Special guidelines for special people: Individuals with hypertension: aim to get no more than 1,500 mg. of sodium per day, and meet the potassium recommendation (4,700 mg./day) with food.*

If you have high blood pressure, then this can be a worthwhile guideline to aim for.

This isn't rocket science. You'll bring your salt intake down just by subbing some fresh fruits for the usual salty snacks. The bottom line is that this is yet another reason to eat your fruits and veggies. Simple stuff like this, along with keeping active, can really lower your blood pressure. Just think of the perks:

- feeling better
- doing more with daily life
- less chance of a stroke or a heart attack
- fewer medications with side effects like sexual dysfunction and lots more

Note the emphasis on getting potassium *from food,* not salt substitutes, supplements, or pills. Salt substitutes are really just potassium chloride. They come in shakers, much like salt, and you can find them in the supermarket right where you get salt.

Salt substitutes don't mix with some medications, and they aren't good for people with some medical conditions, especially people who have certain types of kidney diseases. The same holds true for potassium pills or supplements. You really need clearance from your physician before you use salt substitutes or potassium supplements or pills. One other thing that may keep you from trying salt substitutes: They don't exactly taste like salt. They tend to taste metallic.

If you rely on supplements to meet your potassium needs, you probably aren't getting all the fruits and vegetables and low-fat dairy foods you need, so start right there. Food is powerful health, and it tastes way better than pills. Besides, you'll never get into a pill what you can get from a good, healthy eating style. And aren't you glad? Talk about taking the fun out of life. Personally, I'm glad they haven't figured out how to get healthy eating into a pill. I enjoy my meals too much, and I really want you to have the same pleasures from eating, too.

Guideline: *Overweight adults with chronic diseases and/or on medication: Consult a healthcare provider about weight loss strategies prior to starting a weight-reduction program to ensure appropriate management of other health conditions.*

I'll add here only that you want a *qualified* healthcare provider. The person behind the counter at the health food store doesn't count. Neither does your personal trainer unless he or she is a nurse, physician, or registered dietitian. If you have special health concerns, consult a specialist. Period.

Guideline: *Those who are immunocompromised: Do not eat or drink raw (unpasteurized) milk or any products made from unpasteurized milk, raw or undercooked eggs, or any foods containing raw eggs, raw or undercooked meat or poultry, unpasteurized juices and raw sprouts, raw or undercooked fish or shellfish.*

This is basically the same food guideline given earlier, with one exception: no raw fish or shellfish for this group. You don't have the same defenses as the rest of us and it's harder for you to kill or fight bacteria you ingest. So hold the sushi, please, and stay away from any oyster that isn't cooked. Incidentally, although cooked fish is fine, some restaurants get snooty and ask things like, "How would you like your salmon cooked, Madame? Rare is how the chef suggests." Rare means that it's undercooked. Tell him or her that Monsieur or Madame would like the salmon cooked through, please. The same holds true for beef and lamb. At least go for medium. It might not be rare, but it's not as risky, either, especially since you can't be there to take its temperature, and medium should put you in the safe zone.

Guideline: *Those who are immunocompromised: Only eat certain deli meats and frankfurters that have been reheated to steaming hot.*

Most deli meats and frankfurters are fine most of the time. But some deli meats, especially cured meats and frankfurters, have been associated with outbreaks of a sometimes fatal foodborne illness caused by an organism called *listeria monocytogenes,* commonly known just as listeria. You can still heat these foods *if they are heated to steaming hot*. Our suggestion is, if you really want a frankfurter or deli meat, prepare it yourself so it's steaming hot. That way you know for sure how it was cooked and handled.

### African Americans

Guideline: *People with dark skin: Consume extra vitamin D from vitamin D–fortified foods and/or sunlight.*

No need to bake in the sun to get your vitamin D. But African Americans and others with dark skin, can't make vitamin D as easily. Also, if you live in a cold climate where you have to stay covered up and indoors for the winter, or if you wear sunscreen regularly, you may not get enough sunshine to make enough vitamin D. That's yet another reason to drink milk, mostly low-fat and fat-free milk. It's the best dietary source of vitamin D we have. Next best are multivitamin supplements with vitamin D. This vitamin is a major player in helping you to use the calcium you're getting, so help yourself out and drink your three-a-day of dairy foods.

Guideline: *Special guidelines for special people: Blacks: aim to get no more than 1,500 mg. of sodium per day, and meet the potassium recommendation (4,700 mg./day) with food.*

As we get older, we tend to get more sensitive to the effects of salt. Black folks as a group have a higher incidence of high blood pressure and they tend to be more sensitive to salt than others. They also tend to have diets that are really low in potassium.

If you have high blood pressure, then this can be a worthwhile guideline to aim for. In any case, definitely eat foods with potassium (no pussyfooting here, this is serious—but you'll find it easy to do over time).

This isn't rocket science. You'll bring your salt intake down just by subbing some fresh fruits for the usual salty snacks. The bottom line is that this is yet another reason to eat your fruits and veggies. Simple stuff like this, along with keeping active, can really lower your blood pressure. Just think of the perks:

- feeling better
- doing more with daily life
- less chance of a stroke or a heart attack
- fewer medications with side effects like sexual dysfunction and lots more

Note the emphasis on getting potassium *from food*, not salt substitutes, supplements, or pills. Salt substitutes are really just potassium chloride. They come in shakers, much like salt, and you can find them in the supermarket right where you get salt.

Salt substitutes don't mix with some medications, and they aren't good for people with some medical conditions, especially people who have certain types of kidney diseases. The same holds true for potassium pills or supplements. You really need clearance from your physician before you use salt substitutes or potassium supplements or pills. One other thing that may keep you from trying salt substitutes: They don't exactly taste like salt. They tend to taste metallic.

If you rely on supplements to meet your potassium needs, you probably aren't getting all the fruits and vegetables and low-fat dairy foods you need, so start right there. Food is powerful health, and it tastes way better than pills. Besides, you'll never get into a pill what you can get from a good, healthy eating style. And aren't you glad? Talk about taking the fun out of life. Personally, I'm glad they haven't figured out how to get healthy eating into a pill. I enjoy my meals too much, and I really want you to have the same pleasures from eating, too.

# CHAPTER 6

# Four Weeks of Meal Plans

Now that you know the philosophy behind the Uncle Sam Diet, all you need to follow through is a blueprint. Here are four weeks of sample menus, a day-by-day listing of meals and snacks to get you started. Each day's meal plan contains approximately 2,000 calories, with ideas for pruning the calories down to 1,500 if you'd like to lose weight. Men might be able to lose weight on 2,000 calories, so just eat a little more of each food to keep your weight stable.

# Day 1

**BREAKFAST**
1 cup wheat flakes, 1 cup low-fat milk, 1 cup sliced strawberries (about 8 medium), coffee or tea

**LUNCH**
whole wheat pita sandwich: 2 ounces sliced roast beef, 2 lettuce leaves, 2 slices tomato, 1 tablespoon mayonnaise; ½ cup baby carrots; 1 ounce plantain chips; 1 cup light yogurt

**AFTERNOON SNACK**
1 apple with 2 tablespoons peanut butter

**DINNER**
4 ounces (size of a deck of cards or a computer mouse) broiled sole or light fish, 1 medium baked potato, 1 tablespoon sour cream, 1 small ear corn on the cob, 1 cup raw vegetable salad with 1 tablespoon oil-and-vinegar dressing, ½ cup lemon sorbet

**EVENING SNACK**
1 cup Dr. Keith's Low-Fat Hot Chocolate (page 175). 2 graham crackers

**Nutrition analysis for the day:**

| | | |
|---|---|---|
| Calories: 2,027 | Protein: 92 g | Carbohydrate: 302 g |
| Fat: 62 g | Saturated fat: 21 g | Cholesterol: 132 mg |
| Dietary fiber: 34 g | Sodium: 1,534 mg | |

**For 1,500 calories:** Omit ½ tablespoon mayo and plantain chips from lunch, peanut butter from afternoon snack, and either corn or potato from dinner.

---

# Day 2

---

**BREAKFAST**
egg sandwich: 2 sliced hard-boiled eggs and 1 slice (about 1 ounce) cheddar cheese on 2 slices whole wheat toast/bread, 1 cup cantaloupe, coffee or tea

**LUNCH**
grilled chicken salad: 2 cups mixed greens with ½ cup cherry tomatoes, 1 tablespoon Parmesan cheese, ½ cup diced, grilled chicken breast; 1 small whole-grain roll; 1 orange

**AFTERNOON SNACK**
1 fat-free latte, 1 ounce almonds

**DINNER**
3-ounce turkey burger, medium sweet potato, 1 cup green beans, 2 plums, 1 granola bar

**EVENING SNACK**
2 cups air-popped popcorn with butter-flavor popcorn spray, 1 cup hot low-fat milk with dash of almond extract and sweetener.

**Nutrition analysis for the day:**

| | | |
|---|---|---|
| Calories: 1,981 | Protein: 113 g | Carbohydrate: 218 g |
| Fat: 80 g | Saturated fat: 24 g | Cholesterol: 617 mg |
| Dietary fiber: 29 g | Sodium: 1,731 mg | |

**For 1,500 calories:** Omit 1 egg and cheese from breakfast, almonds from afternoon snack, and milk from evening snack.

# Day 3

**BREAKFAST**
1 cup oatmeal with ¼ cup raisins and 1 cup low-fat milk, 1 banana, coffee or tea

**LUNCH**
light Cobb salad: 1 cup shredded greens, 1 cup steamed broccoli or cauliflower, 1 ounce blue cheese, ½ cup garbanzo beans, 1 ounce chopped almonds, 2 ounces diced turkey breast, 2 tablespoons low-fat blue cheese dressing

**AFTERNOON SNACK**
4 whole wheat crackers, 1 cup grapes

**DINNER**
Mediterranean Braised Beef (page 153) over 1 cup brown rice, 6 asparagus spears, Baked Apple (page 170)

**EVENING SNACK**
1 cup light yogurt, 1 oatmeal cookie

**Nutrition analysis for the day:**

| | | |
|---|---|---|
| Calories: 1,970 | Protein: 102 g | Carbohydrate: 280 g |
| Fat: 55 g | Saturated fat: 12 g | Cholesterol: 181 mg |
| Dietary fiber: 32 g | Sodium: 3,314 mg | |

**For 1,500 calories:** Omit raisins from oatmeal at breakfast, ¼ cup garbanzos and the almonds from lunch, ½ cup of rice from dinner, and substitute a fresh apple for the baked apple at dinner

# Day 4

**BREAKFAST**
1 cup toasted oat cereal (like Cheerios), 1 cup low-fat milk, 1 cup sliced strawberries, coffee or tea

**LUNCH**
toasted cheese sandwich: 2 slices whole wheat bread with 2 one-ounce slices low-fat cheese; 1 cup baby carrots and snap peas, fresh pear

**AFTERNOON SNACK**
2 tablespoons peanut butter; 4 saltines

**DINNER**
linguine with Roasted Garlic Sauce (page 152), 1 cup red pepper and onion salad, 1 tablespoon Italian dressing, 1 slice Italian bread, ½ cup fruit sorbet

**EVENING SNACK**
1 cup milk, 4 Dove Minis

**Nutrition analysis for the day:**

| | | |
|---|---|---|
| Calories: 2,014 | Protein: 82 g | Carbohydrate: 263 g |
| Fat: 78 g | Saturated fat: 21 g | Cholesterol: 43 mg |
| Dietary fiber: 36 g | Sodium: 1,675 mg | |

**For 1,500 calories:** Have half a sandwich at lunch, half the peanut butter at the afternoon snack, omit the Italian bread at dinner, and have only 1 Dove Mini for the evening snack.

# Day 5

**BREAKFAST**
2 scrambled eggs, 1 small bran muffin (2 ounces), 1 cup honeydew chunks, coffee or tea

**LUNCH**
1 ounce lean roast beef, 1 ounce Swiss cheese, 2 slices whole wheat bread, 1 teaspoon mayo, 1 cup mixed fruit salad

## AFTERNOON SNACK
tall nonfat latte (10 ounces), 1 oatmeal cookie

## DINNER
4 ounces grilled salmon, 2 grilled portobello mushrooms with 1 tablespoon Parmesan, 1 ear corn on the cob, 1 cup green salad, 1 tablespoon Italian dressing

## EVENING SNACK
1 cup light yogurt, ¼ cup dried apricots (about 5)

**Nutrition analysis for the day:**

| | | |
|---|---|---|
| Calories: 1,986 | Protein: 102 g | Carbohydrate: 248 g |
| Fat: 74 g | Saturated fat: 21 g | Cholesterol: 653 mg |
| Dietary fiber: 24 g | Sodium: 1,665 mg | |

**For 1,500 calories:** Have only 1 egg at breakfast, ½ cup fruit salad at lunch, omit the oatmeal cookie from the afternoon snack, have fat-free salad dressing at dinner, and omit the raisins from the evening snack.

# Day 6

## BREAKFAST
1 cup raisin bran, 1 cup low-fat milk, 1 banana, 1 slice whole wheat toast, 1 teaspoon trans-free spread, coffee or tea

## LUNCH
minipizza: 1 ounce low-fat mozzarella on each of 2 whole wheat English muffin halves, ¼ cup meatless pasta sauce; ½ cup baby carrots; ½ cup pineapple chunks packed in juice

## AFTERNOON SNACK
1½-ounce box of raisins, 1 ounce almonds

## DINNER
1 baked chicken breast (3 ounces): 1 cup Tabbouleh salad (page 162), 1 cup sliced, broiled zucchini; 1 tablespoon grated Parmesan; 2 cups mixed green salad with 1 tablespoon Italian dressing; 2 sliced kiwi

## EVENING SNACK
1 slice angel food cake (¹⁄₁₂ cake), ½ cup low fat ice cream, 1 tablespoon chocolate syrup

**Nutrition analysis for the day:**

| | | |
|---|---|---|
| Calories: 1,936 | Protein: 98 g | Carbohydrate: 286 g |
| Fat: 56 g | Saturated fat: 16 g | Cholesterol: 153 mg |
| Dietary fiber: 40 g | Sodium: 2,463 mg | |

**For 1,500 calories:** Omit the toast and spread from breakfast, substitute 1 cup of grapes for the afternoon snack, and have fat-free salad dressing at dinner.

# Day 7

**BREAKFAST**
1 ounce smoked salmon, ½ large or 1 small whole wheat bagel (2 ounces), 1 tablespoon cream cheese, 1 cup orange juice, coffee or tea

**LUNCH**
Cowboy Ranch Flank Steak Salad (page 158), 1 whole wheat roll, 1 cup sliced papaya

**AFTERNOON SNACK**
1 cup grape tomatoes, 1 ounce low-fat cheddar cheese, 4 whole wheat crackers

**DINNER**
3 ounces roast turkey breast; mashed roast sweet potato with maple syrup; 1 cup string beans with ½ ounce sliced almonds; 1 glass (5 ounces) wine; 1 apple, cored, sliced, sprinkled with cinnamon and 1 teaspoon sugar

**EVENING SNACK**
1 cup Dr. Keith's Low-Fat Hot Chocolate (page 175), 1 oatmeal cookie

**Nutrition analysis for the day:**

| | | |
|---|---|---|
| Calories: 2,013 | Protein: 110 g | Carbohydrate: 283 g |
| Fat: 49 g | Saturated fat: 14 g | Cholesterol: 154 mg |
| Dietary fiber: 37 g | Sodium: 2,527 mg | |

**For 1,500 calories:** Omit the cream cheese and ½ cup juice from breakfast, the cheese and crackers from the afternoon snack, the wine from dinner, and the cookie from the evening snack.

# Day 8

**BREAKFAST**
1 whole wheat pancake (6-inch) diameter with 1 tablespoon syrup, 1 scrambled egg, 1 cup mixed berries, coffee or tea

**LUNCH**
Grilled Eggplant-Tomato Sandwich (page 164), 1 ounce plantain chips, 1 orange

**AFTERNOON SNACK**
1 tall nonfat latte, 1 banana

**DINNER**
1 baked medium pork chop, 2 small roasted red potatoes, 2 cups mixed greens with 2 tablespoons Italian dressing, ½ cup low-fat ice cream

**EVENING SNACK**
1 ounce dark chocolate, 1 cup milk

**Nutrition analysis for the day:**

| | | |
|---|---|---|
| Calories: 2,006 | Protein: 75 g | Carbohydrate: 273 g |
| Fat: 75 g | Saturated fat: 31 g | Cholesterol: 355 mg |
| Dietary fiber: 31 g | Sodium: 1,794 mg | |

**For 1,500 calories:** Omit the egg from breakfast, the chips from lunch, 1 of the potatoes, and substitute fat-free salad dressing at dinner, and omit the milk in the evening (sometimes you just need some chocolate, even on a diet).

# Day 9

**BREAKFAST**
2 ounces Brie, 1 cup grapes, 6 whole wheat crackers, coffee or tea

**LUNCH**
Whole wheat wrap: 2 ounces turkey breast, 1 whole wheat tortilla (6-inch) diameter, lettuce leaves, cucumber slices, ¼ avocado wedge, 2 teaspoon mustard; 2 tangerines

**AFTERNOON SNACK**
½ cup soft frozen yogurt, 1 ounce almonds

**DINNER**
Ginger scallops (page 151) over 1 cup brown rice–garbanzo pilaf (½ cup brown rice mixed with ½ cup gar-

banzo beans), 2 cups salad greens, 2 tablespoons Italian dressing, ¾-inch wedge watermelon

EVENING SNACK
herb tea, 2 fig newtons

**Nutrition analysis for the day:**

| | | |
|---|---|---|
| Calories: 1,975 | Protein: 88 g | Carbohydrate: 242 g |
| Fat: 80 g | Saturated fat: 20 g | Cholesterol: 148 mg |
| Dietary fiber: 27 g | Sodium: 2,634 mg | |

**For 1,500 calories:** Omit 1 ounce of cheese and 3 crackers from breakfast, the avocado from lunch, the almonds from the afternoon snack, and substitute fat-free salad dressing at dinner.

# Day 10

BREAKFAST
1 cup whole wheat flakes, 1 sliced banana, 1 slice whole wheat toast, 1 tablespoon peanut butter, 1 cup low-fat milk, coffee or tea

LUNCH
grilled salmon salad: 2 ounces salmon over 2 cups mixed greens, 1 tablespoon Italian dressing; 1 whole grain roll; sugar-free beverage

**AFTERNOON SNACK**
Yogurt Smoothie (page 175)

**DINNER**
Beef and Vegetable Skillet (page 159), 8 spears steamed
asparagus, 1 glass (5 ounces) wine, Almond Biscotti
with Almond Cream (page 167)

**EVENING SNACK**
herb tea, ¼ cup peanuts, 1½ ounce box raisins

**Nutrition analysis for the day:**

| | | |
|---|---|---|
| Calories: 2,003 | Protein: 112 g | Carbohydrate: 251 g |
| Fat: 61 g | Saturated fat: 14 g | Cholesterol: 133 mg |
| Dietary fiber: 27 g | Sodium: 1,975 mg | |

**For 1,500 calories:** Omit the toast and peanut butter from breakfast, substitute fat-free dressing at lunch, omit the dinner wine,
and substitute 1 cup fresh peach slices for the dessert at dinner.

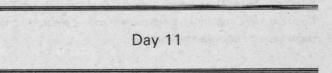

# Day 11

**BREAKFAST**
vegetable omelet: 2 eggs, ½ cup chopped broccoli; 2
slices whole wheat toast; 1 cup orange juice; coffee or
tea

## LUNCH
whole-wheat pita pocket: 1 cup raw veggies (pepper strips, cucumber slices, red onions, 4 sliced olives), ¼ cup crumbled feta cheese: 1 orange

## AFTERNOON SNACK
tall nonfat latte, 3 dates stuffed with walnut halves

## DINNER
Chicken florentine (page 146), 1 cup Oven-Potato Spears (page 165), 1 cup steamed cauliflower (dash of salt), 1 cup fresh sliced strawberries with 1 teaspoon sugar

## EVENING SNACK
1 cup Dr. Keith's Low-Fat Hot Chocolate (page 175)

**Nutrition analysis for the day:**

| | | |
|---|---|---|
| Calories: 1,980 | Protein: 116 g | Carbohydrate: 262 g |
| Fat: 61 g | Saturated fat: 17 g | Cholesterol: 576 mg |
| Dietary fiber: 36 g | Sodium: 2,229 mg | |

**For 1,500 calories:** Omit 1 egg, 1 slice of toast, and ½ cup juice from breakfast, the dates from the afternoon snack, and the sugar from the strawberries at dinner.

# Day 12

**BREAKFAST**
2 slices whole wheat raisin toast, 2 tablespoons peanut butter, 1 cup nonfat yogurt, 1 cup orange sections, coffee or tea

**LUNCH**
1½ cups bean/pepper salad: ½ cup each green beans, garbanzos, chopped red pepper, with 2 tablespoons Italian dressing, 1 tablespoon grated Parmesan; 1 whole-grain roll; 2 plums

**AFTERNOON SNACK**
1 cup low-fat chocolate milk, 1 granola bar

**DINNER**
2 Soft Soy Tacos (page 163), 1 cup sliced cucumbers and onions with 1 tablespoon Italian dressing, 1 cup diced papaya

**EVENING SNACK**
1 slice angel food cake (¹⁄₁₂ cake), ½ cup light ice cream

**Nutrition analysis for the day:**

| | | |
|---|---|---|
| Calories: 1,986 | Protein: 74 g | Carbohydrate: 291 g |
| Fat: 66 g | Saturated fat: 15 g | Cholesterol: 66 mg |
| Dietary fiber: 31 g | Sodium: 3,138 mg | |

For 1,500 calories: Omit 1 slice toast and 1 tablespoon peanut butter from breakfast, substitute fat-free dressing at lunch and dinner, and have only 1 taco at dinner.

# Day 13

## BREAKFAST
½ cantaloupe filled with 1 cup light yogurt (any flavor), 1 slice whole wheat raisin toast, 1 teaspoon transfree margarine, coffee or tea

## LUNCH
salad bowl: 2 ounces poached salmon, 1 cup sliced mushrooms, ½ cup garbanzo beans, 1 cup chopped spinach, 2 tablespoons Italian dressing; 1 whole-grain roll; 1 cup pineapple chunks

## AFTERNOON SNACK
low-fat ice cream cone (1 scoop)

## DINNER
3 ounces roast pork loin, 1 medium baked sweet potato, 1 cup steamed broccoli/cauliflower with 1 tablespoon Parmesan, Pear and Apple Crisp with Cranberries (page 173)

**EVENING SNACK**
1 cup warm milk with sweetener and dash of almond extract, 1 oatmeal cookie

**Nutrition analysis for the day:**

| | | |
|---|---|---|
| Calories: 1,992 | Protein: 88 g | Carbohydrate: 285 g |
| Fat: 53 g | Saturated fat: 14 g | Cholesterol: 114 mg |
| Dietary fiber: 29 g | Sodium: 1,995 mg | |

**For 1,500 calories:** Substitute fat-free dressing at lunch, 1 cup grapes for the afternoon snack, a fresh apple for the dessert at dinner, and omit the cookie from the evening snack.

## Day 14

**BREAKFAST**
1 cup whole-grain oat cereal, 1 cup low-fat milk, ½ grapefruit, coffee or tea

**LUNCH**
2 tablespoons peanut butter and 1 tablespoon jelly on 2 slices whole-grain raisin bread, 1 ounce plantain chips, 1 medium apple

**AFTERNOON SNACK**
1 ounce almonds, sugar-free iced tea

## DINNER
1 small baked chicken breast, 1 medium baked potato with 1 tablespoon sour cream, 1 cup snow peas and mushrooms stir-fried in 2 teaspoons olive oil, 1 cup pepper/jicama/onion salad with 1 tablespoon dressing, 1 glass (5 ounces) wine, 1 pear

## EVENING SNACK
1 cup light yogurt

**Nutrition analysis for the day:**

| | | |
|---|---|---|
| Calories: 1,974 | Protein: 78 g | Carbohydrate: 249 g |
| Fat: 73 g | Saturated fat: 22 g | Cholesterol: 103 mg |
| Dietary fiber: 27 g | Sodium: 1,274 mg | |

**For 1,500 calories:** Omit 1 tablespoon peanut butter and the chips from lunch, substitute an oatmeal cookie for the afternoon snack, and omit the wine from dinner.

# Day 15

## BREAKFAST
1 whole wheat English muffin with 1 ounce cheddar cheese on each half, 1 pear, coffee or tea

## LUNCH
½ cup hummus, 1 whole wheat pita, ½ cup baby carrots, 5 celery sticks, 2 plums

**AFTERNOON SNACK**
1 nonfat latte, 1 ounce dark chocolate

**DINNER**
4 ounces baked salmon, 1 cup brown rice, 1 cup mixed vegetables, 1 cup tomato and onion salad with 1 tablespoon Italian dressing and 1 tablespoon Parmesan

**EVENING SNACK**
1 cup light yogurt (any flavor), 1 ounce almonds

**Nutrition analysis for the day:**

| | | |
|---|---|---|
| Calories: 1,945 | Protein: 91 g | Carbohydrate: 263 g |
| Fat: 67 g | Saturated fat: 18 g | Cholesterol: 95 mg |
| Dietary fiber: 42 g | Sodium: 2,691 mg | |

**For 1,500 calories:** Omit half an English muffin and 1 ounce of the cheese at breakfast, omit ½ cup rice at dinner, and omit the almonds from the evening snack.

# Day 16

**BREAKFAST**
yogurt parfait: 1 cup light yogurt, ½ cup low-fat granola, ½ cup blueberries; 1 slice whole-grain toast; 1 teaspoon trans-free margarine; coffee or tea

## LUNCH

Black Soybean Salad (page 161) sprinkled with ¼ cup grated low-fat cheddar cheese, ½ cup cherry tomatoes, 1 whole-grain roll

## AFTERNOON SNACK

1 cup low-fat chocolate milk, 1 granola bar

## DINNER

Mediterranean Braised Beef (page 153), 1 grilled portobello mushroom, 1 tablespoon grated Parmesan, ½ grilled red pepper, 1 cup brown rice, ½ cup sliced cucumber, 1 scoop low-fat frozen yogurt

## EVENING SNACK

1 apple, 1 tablespoon peanut butter

**Nutrition analysis for the day:**

| | | |
|---|---|---|
| Calories: 1,996 | Protein: 99 g | Carbohydrate: 293 g |
| Fat: 55 g | Saturated fat: 16 g | Cholesterol: 144 mg |
| Dietary fiber: 29 g | Sodium: 2,643 mg | |

**For 1,500 calories:** Omit the cheese from lunch, the granola bar from the afternoon snack, ½ cup rice from dinner, and the peanut butter from the evening snack.

# Day 17

**BREAKFAST**
1 cup shredded wheat, 1 cup low-fat milk, ½ cup orange juice, 1 small banana, coffee or tea

**LUNCH**
1 ounce turkey and 1-ounce slice reduced-fat Swiss cheese on 2 slices whole wheat bread, 1 tablespoon mayo, 1 cup baby carrots

**AFTERNOON SNACK**
1 cup light yogurt with 1 ounce walnuts (about 7)

**DINNER**
Roast Pork Tenderloin with Apple-Walnut Rice (page 155), 1 cup steamed broccoli, 1 tablespoon trans-free margarine, 1 Baked Apple (page 170)

**EVENING SNACK**
2 cups popcorn, ¼ cup raisins

**Nutrition analysis for the day:**

| | | |
|---|---|---|
| Calories: 1,964 | Protein: 86 g | Carbohydrate: 289 g |
| Fat: 62 g | Saturated fat: 13 g | Cholesterol: 135 mg |
| Dietary fiber: 32 g | Sodium: 1,522 mg | |

**For 1,500 calories:** Omit the orange juice from breakfast, the mayo from lunch, the margarine from dinner, and substitute a fresh apple for the baked apple at dinner, and omit the raisins from the evening snack.

---

# Day 18

---

**BREAKFAST**
1 cup raisin bran, 1 cup low-fat milk, 1 cup strawberries, 1 scrambled egg, coffee or tea

**LUNCH**
tuna salad: 2 ounces water-packed tuna (⅓ standard can), 1 tablespoon mayonnaise, 2 slices tomato, 2 slices cucumber; 2 small plums

**AFTERNOON SNACK**
½ small bagel (3-inch diameter), 1 tablespoon peanut butter

**DINNER**
Pepper-Rubbed Shoulder Center Steak (page 154), 1 cup Oven Potato Spears (page 165) 1 cup peas and carrots, 1 cup orange sections

**EVENING SNACK**
½ cup low-fat ice cream, 1 tablespoon chocolate syrup

**Nutrition analysis for the day:**

| | | |
|---|---|---|
| Calories: 2,020 | Protein: 100 g | Carbohydrate: 266 g |
| Fat: 70 g | Saturated fat: 14 g | Cholesterol: 333 mg |
| Dietary fiber: 37 g | Sodium: 1,846 mg | |

**For 1,500 calories:** Omit the egg from breakfast, use fat-free mayonnaise at lunch, substitute 1 ounce whole wheat pretzels (a small handful) or a banana for the afternoon snack, and substitute 1 cup light yogurt for the ice cream for the evening snack.

# Day 19

**BREAKFAST**
1 cup whole wheat flakes, 1 cup low-fat milk, ½ cup orange juice, 1 slice whole wheat toast with 1 teaspoon peanut butter, 1 banana, coffee or tea

**LUNCH**
chicken salad: ½ cup cooked, diced chicken breast, ½ cup diced tomatoes, ½ cup chopped celery, ¼ cup crumbled blue cheese, ½ cup canned pineapple, juice drained, 1 cup shredded lettuce, 2 tablespoons low-fat blue cheese dressing; 6 wheat crackers

**AFTERNOON SNACK**
1 ounce chocolate bar (or about 4 Dove Minis), 1 almond biscotto

**DINNER**
4 ounces broiled cod, 1 broiled portobello mushroom
with 1 tablespoon grated Parmesan, Zucchini with
Walnuts (page 166), 1 ear corn on the cob, 1 tablespoon trans-free margarine, 1 glass (5 ounces) wine, 1
cup fresh pineapple chunks

**EVENING SNACK**
Yogurt Smoothie (page 175)

**Nutrition analysis for the day:**

| | | |
|---|---|---|
| Calories: 1,947 | Protein: 95 g | Carbohydrate: 239 g |
| Fat: 60 g | Saturated fat: 22 g | Cholesterol: 153 mg |
| Dietary fiber: 34 g | Sodium: 2,616 mg | |

**For 1,500 calories:** Omit the juice and peanut butter from breakfast, the blue cheese from lunch, the biscotto from the afternoon snack, the wine from dinner, and the peaches from the
smoothie for the evening snack.

## Day 20

**BREAKFAST**
1 cup oatmeal, 1 banana, 1 cup light yogurt, coffee or tea

**LUNCH**
1 whole wheat English muffin with 1 ounce low-fat
mozzarella and 2 tablespoons tomato paste on each
half, 1 cup red and green pepper slices, 1 orange

**AFTERNOON SNACK**
2 cups air-popped popcorn

**DINNER**
Chipotle-Marinated Beef Flank Steak (page 147), baked potato, 2 tablespoons sour cream, 1 cups tossed salad greens with 1 tablespoon Italian dressing, 1 cup cantaloupe chunks

**EVENING SNACK**
1 cup Dr. Keith's Low-Fat Hot Chocolate (page 175), 1 ounce almonds

**Nutrition analysis for the day:**

| | | |
|---|---|---|
| Calories: 2,013 | Protein: 107 g | Carbohydrate: 285 g |
| Fat: 59 g | Saturated fat: 18 g | Cholesterol: 149 mg |
| Dietary fiber: 43 g | Sodium: 1,781 mg | |

**For 1,500 calories:** Omit 1 ounce cheese and ½ English muffin from lunch, the sour cream from dinner, and substitute fat-free dressing for the dinner salad, and omit the almonds from the evening snack.

# Day 21

**BREAKFAST**
1 cup light yogurt, 1 cup mixed berries, 1 slice whole wheat toast, 1 tablespoon peanut butter, coffee or tea

**LUNCH**
Sandwich: 2 ounces roast beef, 1 tablespoon mayonnaise, 2 slices tomato, 1 leaf romaine lettuce, 1 whole wheat pita pocket; 1 cup baby carrots; 1 orange

**AFTERNOON SNACK**
1 ounce low-fat cheddar cheese, 6 whole wheat crackers, 1 cup grapes

**DINNER**
Sumptuous Salmon Steaks (page 156), 2 cups tossed green salad with 1 tablespoon grated Parmesan and 1 tablespoon Italian dressing, ½ cup steamed broccoli, 1 whole wheat roll

**EVENING SNACK**
¼ cup dried apricots, 1 cup low-fat milk

**Nutrition analysis for the day:**

| | | |
|---|---|---|
| Calories: 1,969 | Protein: 86 g | Carbohydrate: 263 g |
| Fat: 73 g | Saturated fat: 24 g | Cholesterol: 165 mg |
| Dietary fiber: 37 g | Sodium: 2,017 mg | |

**For 1,500 calories:** Omit the peanut butter from breakfast, the mayo from lunch, the crackers from the afternoon snack, omit the roll and use fat-free salad dressing at dinner, and omit the dried apricots from the evening snack.

# Day 22

**BREAKFAST**
1 small bagel (2 ounces), 1 scrambled egg, 1 cup low-fat milk, 1 cup pineapple chunks, fresh or juice-packed, coffee or tea

**LUNCH**
sandwich: 1 ounce smoked turkey, 1 ounce low-fat Swiss cheese, 2 teaspoons mustard, lettuce, 2 slices tomato, 2 slices whole wheat bread; 1 ounce plantain chips; 1 nectarine

**AFTERNOON SNACK**
1 ounce dark chocolate

**DINNER**
¾ cup dry elbow macaroni (1½ cups cooked) with ½ cup edamame and ½ cup meatless pasta sauce, 2 tablespoons Parmesan cheese, 2 cups tossed salad greens with 1 tablespoon dressing, 1 whole-grain roll, 1 glass (5 ounces wine), 1 cup mixed berries

## EVENING SNACK
½ cup sorbet, 2 graham crackers

**Nutrition analysis for the day:**

| | | |
|---|---|---|
| Calories: 2,018 | Protein: 75 g | Carbohydrate: 295 g |
| Fat: 58 g | Saturated fat: 24 g | Cholesterol: 261 mg |
| Dietary fiber: 32 g | Sodium: 2,307 mg | |

**For 1,500 calories:** Omit the egg from breakfast, the chips from lunch, the wine from dinner, and use fat-free dressing at dinner, and substitute 2 cups air-popped popcorn for the evening snack.

# Day 23

## BREAKFAST
1 cup oat cereal, 1 cup low-fat milk, 1 banana, 1 slice whole-grain toast, 1 teaspoon trans-free margarine, coffee or tea

## LUNCH
bean salad: ½ cup kidney beans, ½ cup green beans, 1 cup lettuce leaves, ½ cup diced firm tofu, 2 tablespoons Italian dressing, 1 small whole wheat roll, 1 pear

**AFTERNOON SNACK**
1 cup light yogurt, 1 ounce almonds

**DINNER**
3 ounces broiled/baked chicken breast (remove skin), 1 small baked sweet potato, 6 spears steamed asparagus with 1 teaspoon trans-free margarine, Caramelized Peaches in Sweet Ricotta (page 171)

**EVENING SNACK**
1 cup fat-free hot chocolate

**Nutrition analysis for the day:**

| | | |
|---|---|---|
| Calories: 2,035 | Protein: 103 g | Carbohydrate: 298 g |
| Fat: 59 g | Saturated fat: 15 g | Cholesterol: 133 mg |
| Dietary fiber: 45 g | Sodium: 2,133 mg | |

**For 1,500 calories:** Use fat-free dressing at lunch, omit the yogurt from the afternoon snack, and substitute a fresh peach or nectarine for the dessert at dinner.

## Day 24

**BREAKFAST**
1 ounce Brie, 1 ounce low-fat cheddar, ½ ounce walnuts (about 7 halves), 1 cup grapes, 6 whole wheat crackers, coffee or tea

## LUNCH
2 ounces turkey breast (2 or 3 slices), lettuce, tomato, 1 tablespoon mayonnaise, 2 slices whole wheat bread, 1 cup baby carrots, 1 orange

## AFTERNOON SNACK
10 ounce fat-free latte, 1 ounce dark chocolate

## DINNER
3 ounces broiled salmon, 1 cup steamed broccoli with 1 tablespoon grated Parmesan, 1 small baked potato with 1 tablespoon sour cream, 1 scoop raspberry sorbet

## EVENING SNACK
1 cup light yogurt, 2 cups air-popped popcorn

**Nutrition analysis for the day:**

| | | |
|---|---|---|
| Calories: 1,993 | Protein: 96 g | Carbohydrate: 255 g |
| Fat: 73 g | Saturated fat: 22 g | Cholesterol: 169 mg |
| Dietary fiber: 31 g | Sodium: 2,070 mg | |

**For 1,500 calories:** Omit the Brie or the cheddar and 3 crackers from breakfast, the mayonnaise from lunch (substitute mustard), the latte or the chocolate from the afternoon snack (maybe have tea instead of the latte and keep same volume of food), omit the sour cream and have 1 cup fresh raspberries instead of the sorbet at dinner, and omit the popcorn from the evening snack.

# Day 25

**BREAKFAST**
1 cup raisin bran, 1 cup 1 percent milk, 1 cup berries, 1 slice whole wheat toast, 1 tablespoon peanut butter, coffee or tea

**LUNCH**
½ cup lentil soup, 1 small whole wheat roll, 1 cup light yogurt, 1 small pear

**AFTERNOON SNACK**
1 cup orange juice, 1 ounce walnuts

**DINNER**
1 baked/broiled pork chop, 1 grilled portobello mushroom, 1 cup spaghetti squash with 1 teaspoon butter and 1 tablespoon grated Parmesan, 1 cup tossed green salad with 1 tablespoon Italian dressing, 1 scoop low-fat ice cream

**EVENING SNACK**
1 cup herb tea, ¼ cup dried apricots, 1 oatmeal cookie

**Nutrition analysis for the day:**

| | | |
|---|---|---|
| Calories: 1,982 | Protein: 93 g | Carbohydrate: 284 g |
| Fat: 64 g | Saturated fat: 16 g | Cholesterol: 147 mg |
| Dietary fiber: 41 g | Sodium: 2,049 mg | |

**For 1,500 calories:** Omit the toast and peanut butter from breakfast, the orange juice from the afternoon snack, use fat-free dressing at dinner and substitute a fresh orange for the ice cream, and omit the dried apricots from the evening snack.

---

# Day 26

---

### BREAKFAST
1 small bagel (2 ounces) or whole wheat English muffin with 1 tablespoon light cream cheese and 1 ounce lox, 1 cup orange juice, coffee or tea

### LUNCH
2 cups or more mixed green salad with 1 ounce sliced turkey breast, ¼ cup diced mozzarella, ½ cup cherry tomatoes, 2 tablespoons Italian dressing; 1 small whole-grain roll, 2 tangerines

### AFTERNOON SNACK
1 ounce almonds, 1 cup light yogurt

### DINNER
Curried Shrimp in a Carrot Nest (page 149), 1 cup brown rice, ½ cup green peas, 1 cup sliced pineapple, fresh or packed in juice

### EVENING SNACK
1 cup low-fat chocolate milk, 2 cups popcorn

**Nutrition analysis for the day:**

| | | |
|---|---|---|
| Calories: 2,032 | Protein: 102 g | Carbohydrate: 299 g |
| Fat: 58 g | Saturated fat: 13 g | Cholesterol: 238 mg |
| Dietary fiber: 36 g | Sodium: 2,444 mg | |

**For 1,500 calories:** Omit the cream cheese from breakfast, the roll from lunch, reduce the rice and the pineapple to ½ cup each at dinner, and omit the popcorn from the evening snack.

# Day 27

**BREAKFAST**
1 cup oatmeal, 1 banana, 1½-ounce box raisins, 1 cup low-fat milk, coffee or tea

**LUNCH**
1 large slice pizza (think New York–style pizza shop) or 2 slices other (Pizza Hut), whole wheat crust if possible, with olives and mushrooms, if desired, 1 apple, sugar-free beverage

**AFTERNOON SNACK**
1 cup sliced fresh or frozen peaches, 1 cup light yogurt

**DINNER**
3 ounces grilled/broiled top round steak, ½ cup brown rice, ½ cup red beans with ¼ cup pasta sauce, 1 cup

(about 5 strips) grilled zucchini, 1 glass (5 ounces) wine, 1 cup strawberries with 1 teaspoon sugar

**EVENING SNACK**
1 ounce bar dark chocolate with almonds (or 4 Dove Minis)

**Nutrition analysis for the day:**

| | | |
|---|---|---|
| Calories: 2,006 | Protein: 98 g | Carbohydrate: 306 g |
| Fat: 41 g | Saturated fat: 19 g | Cholesterol: 130 mg |
| Dietary fiber: 39 g | Sodium: 2,685 mg | |

**For 1,500 calories:** Omit the raisins from breakfast, the yogurt from the afternoon snack, the beans and the wine from dinner (this time the chocolate trumps the beans—not in nutrition, just for pleasure).

# Day 28

**BREAKFAST**
2-egg omelet with ½ cup chopped broccoli (or leftover veggies from the night before), 1 cup diced honeydew melon, 2 slices whole-grain toast, 2 teaspoons trans-free margarine, coffee or tea

**LUNCH**
whole wheat pita stuffed with 2 ounces water-packed tuna (⅓ of standard can), 1 tablespoon mayo, 1 cup

chopped lettuce, tomatoes, cucumbers, scallions; 2 tangerines; bottled water or sugar-free drink

### AFTERNOON SNACK
fat-free latte, 1 ounce M & Ms (fills an empty Velamints tin)

### DINNER
Brown Rice and Chicken Skillet Dinner (page 145), 1 cup 3-bean salad (commercially made is fine), 1 apple, 2 tablespoons peanut butter

### EVENING SNACK
1 cup light yogurt, 1 low-fat granola bar (1 ounce)

**Nutrition analysis for the day:**

| | | |
|---|---|---|
| Calories: 1,985 | Protein: 95 g | Carbohydrate: 249 g |
| Fat: 76 g | Saturated fat: 21 g | Cholesterol: 515 mg |
| Dietary fiber: 31 g | Sodium: 2,156 mg | |

**For 1,500 calories:** Omit 1 egg, 1 slice of toast, and 1 teaspoon margarine from breakfast, the peanut butter from dinner, and the granola bar from the evening snack.

# CHAPTER 7

# The Recipes

I'd love to take complete credit for all the recipes included in the Uncle Sam Diet, but I can't. I like to play around with recipes sometimes, and I include some recipes that have been in the family for a while.

The Uncle Sam Diet is all about variety. That's why the recipes here really run the gamut. There's everything here from beef and pork, to soybeans and nuts. And I'd never forget dessert.

To get the best recipes, I went to experts in their fields. Where better to get a really good beef recipe than the beef guys, the National Cattlemen's Beef Association? The USA Rice Federation has a ton of recipes with all kinds of rice dishes for every part of the meal, from appetizers straight through to dessert. Uncle Sam isn't a total carnivore, though, and the United Soybean Board comes through with some excellent light dishes that please even the most stubborn palate. The Produce for Better Health Foundation is where it's at for exciting ways to get more fruits and vegetables into everyone (yes, even the men). And Graham Kerr developed a fantastic dessert for the Almond

Board of California. Full disclosure: No one paid to get their recipes in here. The goal was simply recipes that were easy and tasty, and would go well with the Uncle Sam Diet.

Great as these recipes are, they're just a start and there are plenty more where they came from. Just go to the Web sites of these organizations:

- Almond Board of California:
  www.almondsarein.com
- National Cattlemen's Beef Association:
  www.beefitswhatsfordinner.com
- Produce for Better Health Foundation:
  www.5aday.com
- USA Rice Federation: www.usarice.com
- United Soybean Board: www.talksoy.com

There are many other commodity board associations. The Uncle Sam Diet includes plenty of low-fat dairy foods, for example, mostly in simple form. The American Dairy Association, for example, has more terrific recipes for all kinds of dairy foods, including lots of low-fat options for drinks, snacks, and main dishes, than you'd ever think possible. Find them at www.3aday.com.

## BROWN RICE AND CHICKEN SKILLET DINNER
**Serves 8**

1 tablespoon oil
1 large onion, chopped
2 large cloves garlic, minced
1 pound boneless, skinless chicken breast, cut
  into 1-inch pieces
1 can (14½ ounces) whole tomatoes, coarsely
  chopped
1 can (6 ounces) tomato paste
½ cup water
2 teaspoons dried Italian seasoning
¼ teaspoons crushed red pepper flakes
3 cups hot cooked brown rice
1 package frozen chopped spinach (10 ounces),
  thawed and squeezed dry
½ cup grated Parmesan cheese

1. Heat oil in large skillet over medium-high heat. Add onion and garlic, and cook 2–3 minutes, or until onion is tender.

2. Add chicken and cook just until chicken loses its pink color, stirring constantly. Add tomatoes, tomato paste, water, Italian seasoning, and pepper flakes.

3. Bring to a boil. Reduce heat and simmer uncovered 5 minutes. Stir in rice, spinach, and ¼ cup Parmesan; heat thoroughly. Sprinkle with remaining ¼ cup cheese just before serving.

**Nutrition information per serving:** 228 calories, 20 g protein, 26 g carbohydrate, 3 g dietary fiber, 6 g fat, 2 g saturated fat, 40 mg cholesterol, 252 mg sodium

*Recipe courtesy of the USA Rice Federation*

## CHICKEN FLORENTINE
Serves 4 (2 cups each)

> 4 cups firmly packed baby spinach leaves, washed, stems removed, or 1 package (10 ounces) frozen, chopped spinach
> 1 teaspoon dried thyme leaves, or 2 teaspoons fresh
> 1 tablespoon olive oil
> 2 cloves garlic, chopped
> ½ cup finely chopped onion
> 1 tablespoon flour
> 1 cup low-sodium chicken broth
> Salt and pepper to taste
> 4 grilled or roasted chicken breasts, shredded or chopped
> 2 lemons, to yield 2 tablespoons grated lemon peel and 4 lemon wedges for garnish

1. Preheat oven to 300°F.

2. Place spinach in a large skillet over medium heat and cook, covered, until fresh is wilted or frozen is heated through. Spinach should have a dark, rich green color. Do not overcook. Remove spinach and drain well.

3. In the same skillet, heat thyme with oil, garlic, and onion, and sauté until onion is transparent. Stir in flour until it disappears. Add broth and stir continuously until a thickened sauce is formed. Return spinach to sauce and mix well. Heat and adjust seasonings, if desired.

4. Stir half the chicken into sauce. To serve, spoon equal amounts in four small casseroles. Top each with equal portions of remaining chicken and ½ tablespoon grated lemon peel. Bake in oven for 10 minutes. Serve piping hot with a lemon wedge.

Note: This is a perfect recipe for leftover cooked chicken, or even extras that were grilled on a previous day.

Nutrition information per serving: 220 calories, 30 g protein, 8 g carbohydrate, 3 g dietary fiber, 7 g fat, 1.5 g saturated fat, 75 mg cholesterol, 150 mg sodium

*Recipe developed for the Produce for Better Health Foundation by Carmen I. Jones, CCP. All 5-A-Day recipes meet nutrition standards that maintain fruits and vegetables as healthy foods.*

CHIPOTLE-MARINATED BEEF FLANK STEAK
Serves 4–6

Marinade
⅓ cup fresh lime juice
¼ cup chopped fresh cilantro
1 tablespoon packed brown sugar

   2 teaspoons minced chipotle chilies in adobo
      sauce
   2 tablespoons adobo sauce (from chilies)
   2 cloves garlic, minced
   1 teaspoon freshly grated lime peel
   1 beef flank steak (about 1½–2 pounds) or beef top
      round steak, cut 1 inch thick (about 1¾ pounds)
   salt

1. Combine marinade ingredients in bowl and mix
well. Place beef steak and marinade in food-safe plastic bag; turn steak to coat. Close bag securely and marinate in refrigerator 6 hours or overnight.

2. Remove steak from marinade; discard marinade.
Place steak on grid over medium, ash-covered coals.
Grill flank steak, uncovered, 17–21 minutes for
medium rare to medium doneness (top round steak
16–18 minutes for medium rare doneness; do not overcook), turning occasionally. Carve steak across the
grain into thin slices. Season with salt, as desired

**Nutrition information per serving, using flank (¼ of recipe): 275
calories, 35 g protein, 3 g carbohydrate, 0 g dietary fiber, 13 g
fat, 4 g saturated fat, 85 mg cholesterol, 124 mg sodium**

*Recipe courtesy of the Cattlemen's Beef Board and the
National Cattlemen's Beef Association.*

## CURRIED SHRIMP IN A CARROT NEST
Serves 4 (1½ cups each)

2 cups coarsely shredded or julienne carrots
1 extra large onion, chopped to yield 2 cups;
   reserve 2 tablespoons
2 tablespoons sugar
1 tablespoon water
2 cups cooked rice, tossed with ½ cup cooked peas
   and 2 tablespoons chopped peanuts, optional
2 tablespoons olive or cooking oil
2 large cloves of garlic, chopped
1 pound peeled medium shrimp (fresh or frozen)
2–3 teaspoons milk curry powder (if spicier is
   desired, use hot curry powder)
2 tablespoons flour
1 cup low-sodium chicken broth
1 tablespoon nonfat yogurt
1 tablespoon lime juice
salt and pepper to taste
1 tablespoon chopped parsley

1. Place shredded carrots, 2 tablespoons chopped onion, and sugar in a medium-sized skillet with 1 tablespoon water. Heat covered, on high to boiling. Cook for 1–2 minutes, until carrots are barely done. Remove immediately and cool.

2. Prepare optional rice suggestion and reserve, if desired.

3. Heat oil in large deep skillet on medium-high heat. Add garlic and peeled shrimp and sauté until shrimp

are opaque and tender. Do not overcook. Remove shrimp from skillet and set aside.

4. To remaining oil in pan, add curry powder and remaining chopped onion. Sauté over medium heat until onions are transparent, coated with curry powder, and somewhat caramelized. Add flour and stir until flour disappears.

5. Add chicken broth and stir continuously until onion curry sauce has thickened. Stir in yogurt, lime juice, and cooked shrimp. Season with salt and pepper if desired.

6. Warm carrots briefly in pan. Place optional rice mixture in large circle on serving plate. Arrange warm carrots inside the ring, and place the curried shrimp in the center. Garnish with chopped parsley. Serve immediately.

**Nutrition information per serving:** 310 calories, 27 g protein, 29 g carbohydrate, 5 g dietary fiber, 10 g fat, 1.5 g saturated fat, 175 mg cholesterol, 230 mg sodium

*Recipe developed for the Produce for Better Health Foundation. All 5-A-Day recipes meet nutrition standards that maintain fruits and vegetables as healthy foods.*

## GINGER SCALLOPS
Serves 4

1½ pounds fresh scallops
3 tablespoons vegetable oil
1½ cups finely chopped celery (include the
   leaves for flavor)
2 cloves garlic
2 tablespoons minced fresh ginger root (more or
   less to taste)
½ cup parsley, finely chopped
¼ teaspoon salt

1. In a large nonstick skillet, heat 2 tablespoons of the oil. When hot, add the scallops and sauté, stirring, for about 3 minutes. They're done when they turn from translucent to opaque. Don't overcook or they'll be tough. Remove to a side dish, keeping as much of the oil and liquid as you can.

2. Add the remaining oil to the skillet and heat. Add celery, garlic, and ginger, and cook until the celery is crisp-tender, then stir in the parsley and the salt.

3. Return the scallops to the skillet and stir to mix. Serve immediately.

**Nutrition information per serving:** 253 calories, 29 g protein, 7 g carbohydrate, 12 g fat, 1.5 g saturated fat, 56 mg cholesterol, 455 mg sodium, 1 g dietary fiber

## LINGUINE WITH ROASTED GARLIC SAUCE
Serves 4

1 head garlic, skin attached (may substitute
  ¼ teaspoon garlic powder and add with the
  chicken broth)
2 teaspoons plus 2 tablespoons soybean oil or
  vegetable oil
8 ounces linguine, fresh or dry
3 tablespoons minced shallots
½ cup dry white wine
½ cup chicken or vegetable broth
2 medium tomatoes, seeded and diced
1 cup edamame (whole green soybeans), shelled
  and cooked
½ cup pine nuts, toasted
¼ cup basil, fresh, chopped, or 1 tablespoon dried
  basil
¼ cup grated Parmesan

1. Preheat the oven to 400°F.

2. Cut pointed top off garlic head, leaving cloves intact, and place on square of aluminum foil. Drizzle 2
teaspoons oil over cloves. Seal foil around garlic and
bake for 30–40 minutes, or until cloves are soft. Cool.
Squeeze paste from cloves, mash, and set aside.

3. Prepare linguine as directed on package. Drain and
set aside.

4. Heat 2 tablespoons oil in a medium saucepan. Add
shallots and garlic paste. Sauté until shallots are
translucent, stirring occasionally.

5. Add wine and broth. Bring to boil and simmer until reduced in half.

6. Add tomatoes and edamame. Cook 1 minute until warmed, stirring gently. Remove from heat. Stir in pine nuts and basil. Add salt and pepper to taste. Spoon over linguine and sprinkle with Parmesan.

**Nutrition information per serving:** 380 calories, 14 g protein, 29 g carbohydrate, 22 g fat, less than 5 mg cholesterol, 250 mg sodium, 6 g dietary fiber

*Recipe courtesy of the United Soybean Board.*

MEDITERRANEAN BRAISED BEEF
Serves 8

    1 boneless beef chuck shoulder pot roast
        (2½–3 pounds)
    ¼ cup all-purpose flour
    2 tablespoons olive oil
    1½ cups water
    ¼ cup balsamic vinegar
    2 small onions, halved and sliced
    4 medium shallots, sliced
    ¼ cup chopped pitted dates
    ½ teaspoon salt
    ¼–½ teaspoon pepper

1. Preheat the oven to 325°F.

2. Lightly coat pot roast with flour. Heat oil in Dutch oven over medium heat until hot. Brown pot roast. Remove.

3. Add the water and vinegar to Dutch oven. Cook and stir until brown bits attached to pan are dissolved. Return pot roast. Add onions, shallots, dates, salt and pepper. Bring to a boil. Cover tightly and cook in the oven oven 2–2½ hours, or until pot roast is fork-tender. Remove pot roast and keep warm.

4. Cook liquid and vegetables over medium-high heat to desired consistency.

5. Carve pot roast. Serve with sauce.

**Nutrition information per serving:** 329 calories, 36 g protein, 16 g carbohydrate, 13 g fat, 270 mg sodium, 110 mg cholesterol

*Recipe courtesy of the Cattlemen's Beef Board and the National Cattlemen's Beef Association.*

## PEPPER-RUBBED SHOULDER CENTER STEAK
Serves 4

  1 teaspoon cracked black pepper or mixed cracked
    peppercorns (black, white, green, and pink)
  1 teaspoon minced garlic
  4 beef shoulder center steaks, ¾ inch thick
    (about 5 ounces each)
  2 teaspoons vegetable oil
  ½ cup beef broth (salt added)
  ¼ cup dry red wine

1. Combine pepper and garlic. Press evenly onto beef steaks.

2. Heat oil in large nonstick skillet over medium heat until hot. Place steaks in skillet and cook 9–11 minutes for medium rare to medium doneness, turning once. Remove to platter and keep warm.

3. Add broth and wine to skillet; increase heat to medium-high. Cook, stirring, 1–2 minutes, or until browned bits attached to skillet are dissolved and sauce is reduced by half.

4. Spoon sauce over steaks.

**Nutrition information per serving:** 215 calories, 29 g protein, 1 g carbohydrate, 2 g dietary fiber, 9 g fat, 1 g saturated fat, 71 mg cholesterol, 182 mg sodium

*Recipe courtesy of the Cattlemen's Beef Board and the National Cattlemen's Beef Association.*

ROAST PORK TENDERLOIN WITH APPLE-WALNUT RICE
Serves 6

　　1 cup rice (white or brown)
　　¼ teaspoon ground white pepper
　　1–1¼ cup water
　　½ cup dry white wine
　　½ cup apple juice
　　1 tablespoon butter or margarine
　　⅔ cup chopped, cored apple
　　½ cup walnuts, chopped
　　1⅓ pounds pork tenderloin, roasted and sliced

1. Combine rice, pepper, water (1 cup water for white rice, 1¼ cup for brown rice), wine, apple juice, and butter saucepan. Bring to a boil; stir once or twice.

2. Reduce heat, cover, and simmer 15 minutes for white rice, 45–50 minutes for brown rice, or until rice is tender and liquid is absorbed.

3. Add apple and walnuts. Fluff with fork. Serve with roasted pork tenderloin slices.

**Nutrition information per serving:** 348 calories, 24 g protein, 32 g carbohydrate, 1 g dietary fiber, 12 g fat, 3 g saturated fat, 71 mg cholesterol, 70 mg sodium

*Recipe courtesy of the USA Rice Federation*

SUMPTUOUS SALMON STEAKS
Serves 2

    2 salmon steaks, 1–1½ inches thick (about 4
      ounces each)
    3 tablespoons butter or margarine
    salt (optional)
    ground black pepper
    1 lime, thinly sliced
    ½ cup coarsely chopped tart red apple
    2 pineapple slices, cut into chunks, with 2
      tablespoons juice
    ½ cup chicken broth
    1½ teaspoon cornstarch
    1 teaspoon sugar

1 cup hot cooked rice
1 tablespoon slivered almonds, toasted

1. Brush salmon steaks with 1 tablespoon melted butter or margarine. Season with salt and pepper, and with juice from the ends of the lime.

2. Place salmon on broiler pan. Broil 3–4 inches from heat source until browned, 4–5 minutes on each side.

3. Meanwhile, melt remaining 2 tablespoons butter or margarine in medium skillet. Add apple and pineapple. Cook over medium heat for 3 minutes.

4. Combine pineapple juice, broth, cornstarch, and sugar. Add to skillet: Cook, stirring, until clear and thickened, 3–5 minutes. Add lime slices. Salt to taste. Serve sauce over salmon and beds of fluffy rice. Garnish with almonds.

**Nutrition information per serving:** 508 calories, 27 g protein, 41 g carbohydrate, 1 g dietary fiber, 27 g fat, 12 g saturated fat, 88 mg cholesterol, 668 mg sodium

*Recipe courtesy of the USA Rice Federation.*

## COWBOY RANCH FLANK STEAK SALAD
Serves 6

Marinade
½ cup Hidden Valley Original Ranch Dressing,
    Light
1 teaspoon chili powder
½ teaspoon onion powder
½ teaspoon garlic powder
½ teaspoon cumin

1 beef flank steak, 1½ pounds
olive oil cooking spray
2 teaspoons garlic herb seasoning (no salt)
1 package (ten ounces) romaine lettuce (about 8
    cups)
6 tablespoons Hidden Valley Original Ranch
    Dressing, Light
8 red potatoes with skin, 2-inch size
1½ cups halved red seedless grapes
2 tablespoons chopped fresh basil
30 croutons
fresh black pepper, to taste

1. Combine marinade ingredients in a small bowl; mix
well. Place beef steak and marinade in food-safe plastic bag, turn steak to coat. Close bag securely and marinate in refrigerator 6 hours or overnight.

2. Preheat oven to 400°F. Wash and cut potatoes into
quarters. Spread evenly on a baking sheet and spray
with olive oil for 3 seconds. Season with garlic herb
seasoning. Roast potatoes in oven for 30 minutes.

3. Remove beef steak from marinade; discard marinade. Place steak on grill over medium, ash-covered coals. Grill flank steak, uncovered, 17–21 minutes for medium rare to medium doneness, turning occasionally. Carve steak across the grain into thin slices.

4. Combine romaine lettuce with Hidden Valley Original Ranch Dressing, Light. Place equal amounts of lettuce mixture on 6 large plates. Add ⅙ of sliced steak to each plate. Distribute potatoes, grape halves, basil, croutons, and black pepper evenly to the 6 plates. Serve immediately.

**Nutritional information per serving:** 423 calories, 31 g protein, 51 g carbohydrate, 11 g fat, 3 g saturated fat, 39 mg cholesterol, 299 mg sodium, 6 g dietary fiber

*Recipe developed for the Produce for Better Health Foundation by Mark Goodwin CEC, CND. All 5-A-Day recipes meet nutrition standards that maintain fruits and vegetables as healthy foods.*

BEEF AND VEGETABLE SKILLET
Serves 4

   1¼ pounds boneless beef top sirloin steak, cut ¾
     inch thick
   2 teaspoons dark sesame oil
   2 garlic cloves, minced
   1 medium red bell pepper, cut into thin strips
   3 tablespoons reduced-sodium soy sauce

2 tablespoons water
3 cups coarsely chopped fresh spinach
½ cup sliced green onions
3 tablespoons ketchup
2 cups hot cooked rice, prepared without butter
   or salt

1. Cut beef steak lengthwise in half and then cross-wise into ¼ inch strips. Toss with sesame oil and garlic.

2. Heat large nonstick skillet over medium-high heat until hot. Add beef (half at a time) and stir-fry 1–2 minutes, or until outside surface is no longer pink. Remove from skillet.

3. In same skillet, add bell pepper, 2 tablespoons soy sauce, and water: Cook 2–3 minutes, or until pepper is crisp-tender. Add spinach and green onions, and cook until spinach is just wilted. Stir in ketchup, remaining 1 tablespoon soy sauce, and beef. Heat through. Serve over rice.

**Nutritional information per serving:** 362 calories, 31 g protein, 38 g carbohydrate, 2 g dietary fiber, 9 g fat, 751 mg sodium, 76 mg cholesterol

*Recipe courtesy of the Cattlemen's Beef Board and the National Cattlemen's Beef Association.*

**BLACK SOYBEAN SALAD**
Serves 6

1 can (16 ounces) black soybeans, drained and
  rinsed
1 cup canned or cooked corn kernels, drained
1 cup sliced celery
½ cup diced sweet red peppers
½ cup diced green peppers
¼ cup sliced green onions
¼ cup olives
2 tablespoons seeded and diced pickled hot
  yellow peppers
¼ cup soybean oil (or vegetable oil)
¼ cup white wine vinegar
¾ teaspoon salt
½ teaspoon chili powder
freshly ground pepper to taste

1. Combine soybeans, corn, celery, peppers, green onions, olives, and hot peppers in a large bowl. Toss to mix.

2. Combine remaining ingredients in a small bowl and whisk to blend, or in a cruet and shake until blended.

3. Pour dressing over soybean mixture and marinate in refrigerator at least 1 hour.

**Nutrition information per serving:** 180 calories, 7 g protein, 16 g carbohydrates, 5 g dietary fiber, 11 g fat, 0 mg cholesterol, 983 mg sodium

*Recipe courtesy of the United Soybean Board.*

## TABBOULEH SALAD

- 1 cup fine bulgur (coarse is too big)
- 2 tomatoes, diced small
- 2 cups chopped parsley (not too fine, and not too loosely packed)
- 4–5 scallions, chopped, use white and most of green top
- 1 small or ½ large cucumber, peeled and diced small
- 3 tablespoons chopped fresh mint (or 2 teaspoons dried, but the fresh is really good)
- 2 teaspoons salt
- ¼ cup olive oil
- ¼ cup fresh lemon juice

1. Put bulgur in a bowl and cover with water. Let sit for about ½ hour. Drain in a fine strainer, pressing to get out excess water. Grain should be moistened but able to be "fluffed."

2. Put soaked bulgur into separate bowl and add rest of ingredients except oil and lemon juice. Toss mixture.

3. Whisk together oil and lemon juice. Pour over salad and refrigerate well. Toss again before serving.

Note: Experiment adding different ingredients, like ½ cup garbanzo beans or diced celery, or ¼ cup slivered almonds.

**Nutrition information per serving:** 191 calories, 4 g protein, 2 g carbohydrate, 10 g fat, 1 g saturated fat, 0 mg cholesterol, 215 mg sodium, 6 g dietary fiber

## SOFT SOY TACOS
Makes 12 tacos

¾ cup boiling water
1 cup texturized soy protein (TSP)
½ pound lean ground beef
½ cup onions, chopped
1 teaspoon soybean oil (vegetable oil)
1 cup tomato sauce
½ cup canned diced green chilies
1 teaspoon chili powder
1 teaspoon garlic salt
¼ teaspoon ground pepper
12 corn tortillas
¾ quart shredded lettuce
1½ cups fresh tomatoes, diced
1½ cups low-fat cheddar cheese
¾ quart salsa, prepared

1. Pour boiling water over TSP.

2. Sauté ground beef and onions in oil until beef is no longer pink. Add rehydrated TSP, tomato sauce, green chilies, chili powder, garlic salt, and pepper. Mix well. Bring mixture to boil, then reduce heat and simmer 15 minutes.

3. Wrap a tortilla in clean towel and microwave at high (100 percent power) 20–25 seconds. Place tortilla on serving plate, spoon ⅓ cup filling in center. Top with ¼ cup shredded lettuce and 2 tablespoons each tomatoes and cheese. Fold in half. Serve with 2 ounces (¼ cup) salsa.

**Nutrition information per taco:** 149 calories, 10 g protein, 16 g carbohydrates, 1.5 g dietary fiber, 4.8 g fat, 1 g saturated fat, 16.2 mg cholesterol, 560 mg sodium

*Recipe courtesy of the United Soybean Board*

GRILLED EGGPLANT-TOMATO SANDWICHES
Serves 4

    1 medium Italian eggplant, unpeeled, cut into
       ½-inch slices
    1 tablespoon salt
    1½ tablespoons olive oil
    2 cloves garlic, crushed
    3 tablespoons finely minced fresh basil
    4 ripe, medium tomatoes
    fresh ground black pepper
    8 half-inch-thick slices of crusty bread
    ½ cup crumbled feta cheese (optional)

1. Sprinkle eggplant on both sides with salt and allow to rest for 10 minutes. Thoroughly rinse slices to remove all salt and drain on paper towel.

2. Combine olive oil and garlic, and lightly brush the mixture on each slice of the eggplant. Grill over

medium-high heat on gas grill or broil under broiler. When soft, remove immediately and sprinkle with basil. Meanwhile, slice tomatoes into ⅓-inch-thick slices and season with black pepper.

3. Arrange tomatoes and eggplant on 4 slices of bread. Season with pepper and add crumbled feta cheese, if desired. Top with second slice of bread and serve immediately.

**Nutrition information per serving (not including optional feta): 260 calories, 7 g protein, 41 g carbohydrate, 8 g fat, 2 g saturated fat, 0 mg cholesterol, 360 mg sodium, 6 gm dietary fiber**

*Recipe developed for the Produce for Better Health Foundation. All 5-A-Day recipes meet nutrition standards that maintain fruits and vegetables as healthy foods.*

OVEN POTATO SPEARS
Serves 4

    4 medium baking potatoes (about 2½–3 inches
       across), washed and scrubbed
    1 tablespoon cooking oil, or several seconds of
       cooking spray
    herbs to taste (garlic or onion powder, chili
       powder, rosemary), if desired.
    ¼ teaspoon seasoned salt

1. Preheat the oven to 350°F.

2. Cut potatoes lengthwise into thick spears (think steak fries).

3. Place the potatoes and oil in a self-seal plastic bag (or place the potatoes in a large bowl and spray with cooking spray two or three times, tossing between sprays). Add desired seasonings salt and toss again.

4. Spread the potatoes onto a large cookie sheet sprayed with cooking spray and bake about 30 minutes, or until desired degree of doneness. Check after 20 minutes to make sure smaller fries don't burn.

**Nutrition information per serving:** 198 calories, 5 g protein, 37 g carbohydrate, 4 g dietary fiber, 4 g fat, .5 g saturated fat, 0 mg cholesterol, 159 mg sodium

## ZUCCHINI WITH WALNUTS
Serves 4 (1¼ cup each)

    4 medium zucchini, washed, stems removed
    ½ tablespoon olive oil
    1 teaspoon walnut oil (optional)
    1 tablespoon coarsely chopped walnuts
    1 teaspoon dried thyme leaves, crushed (or 2
        teaspoons fresh thyme leaves)
    1 lemon, grated peel and juice
    ½ teaspoon salt
    black pepper, to taste

1. Cut zucchini in quarters lengthwise and then into ¾-inch chunks.

2. Heat oil(s) in a 10-inch skillet over medium-high heat. Add zucchini and sauté, stirring constantly and gently.

3. When zucchini is almost tender, add walnuts and thyme, and continue to cook for about 45–60 seconds. Zucchini should still be bright green in color. Season with lemon juice, grated lemon peel, salt, and pepper. Serve hot.

Notes: Walnut oil is available in specialty food shops and select grocery stores. It turns rancid quickly, so store between uses in an airtight container in the refrigerator.

Nutrition information per serving: 100 calories, 4 g protein, 20 g carbohydrate, 6 g dietary fiber, 4 g fat, 1 g saturated fat, 0 mg cholesterol, 290 mg sodium

*Recipe developed for the Produce for Better Health Foundation by Carmen I. Jones, CCP. All 5-A-Day recipes meet nutrition standards that maintain fruits and vegetables as healthy foods.*

## ALMOND BISCOTTI WITH ALMOND CREAM
Serves 4

Almond Biscotti
2 tablespoons extra light olive oil
½ cup chopped, blanched almonds
2 cups flour
2 teaspoons baking powder

¼ teaspoon salt
½ cup brown sugar
2 tablespoons honey
¼ cup egg substitute
½ teaspoon vanilla extract
½ teaspoon almond extract

Almond Cream
1 cup evaporated skim milk
1 cup 2 percent milk
¼ cup sugar
½ teaspoon almond extract
½ teaspoon vanilla extract
1 cup egg substitute
4 Almond Biscotti (recipe below)
2 tablespoons roasted sliced almonds
½ teaspoon instant espresso coffee or finely
   ground espresso coffee

Almond Biscotti

1. Preheat the oven to 350°F.

2. Oil a large baking sheet and arrange almonds in a single layer. Roast the almonds 5–8 minutes, or until golden brown. Almonds will darken and become fragrant. Set aside to cool. (Don't turn off the oven.)

3. Combine the flour, baking powder, and salt in a small bowl.

4. Beat together the brown sugar, honey, egg substitute, and vanilla and almond extracts with an electric

mixer. Add the flour mixture and beat until mixed. Stir in the almonds.

5. Divide the dough and form into two balls. Roll each ball into a 10" cylinder and place them on the baking sheet 5 inches apart. Bake for 20–25 minutes, or until the top is golden brown and slightly cracked. Cool on a rack until just barely warm.

6. Place the cooled rolls on a cutting board and cut on the diagonal into ½-inch slices. Place the slices back on the baking sheet and bake 10–12 minutes more. Cool on a wire rack.

Makes 20 biscotti

### Almond Cream

1. Combine the evaporated skim milk, 2 percent milk, sugar, and almond and vanilla extracts in a heavy saucepan or top of a double boiler. Heat, stirring, on medium high until bubbles form around the edge of the pan.

2. Pour in the egg substitute, whisking vigorously. Cook, stirring constantly, until the mixture thickens and coats the back of a wooden spoon. Cook just until as thick as heavy cream. Overcooking will result in scrambled eggs!

3. Place the almond biscotti in 4 dessert dishes. Pour the warm custard cream over the top and let sit for a few minutes to soften. It's even better chilled.

4. Combine the roasted almonds and coffee and scatter over the top.

Note: The roasted, sliced almonds, combined with a few instant coffee crystals is wonderful on low-fat ice cream, yogurt, poached pears, peaches, and other stone fruits.

Nutrition information, per biscotto: 102 calories, 2 g protein, 14 g carbohydrate, 1 g dietary fiber, 4 g fat, .5 g saturated fat, 0 mg cholesterol, 66 mg sodium

Nutrition information per serving of whole dessert: 243 calories, 17 g protein, 26 g carbohydrates, 1 g fiber, 7 g fat, 2 g saturated fat, 7 mg cholesterol, 281 mg sodium

*Recipe developed by Graham Kerr for the Almond Board of California.*

BAKED APPLES
Serves 4

    4 medium-sized tart, crisp apples (fuji apples are
       great for this, or red delicious, pippins, or
       Granny Smiths)
    ¼ cup dark brown sugar
    ¼ cup raisins
    cinnamon
    1 tablespoon trans-free margarine
    1 cup apple juice

1. Preheat the oven to 350°F.

2. Peel just the top of the apples, about an inch all around. Core the apples but keep the bottoms intact so the filling stays put.

3. Stuff each apple with 1 tablespoon of brown sugar and 1 tablespoon of raisins. Sprinkle with cinnamon to taste. Dot with margarine and place in an 8- or 9-inch square nonaluminum baking dish.

4. Bake for about 45 minutes, or until tender. Baste with the apple juice and drizzle more juice before serving.

**Nutrition information per serving:** 225 calories, 1 g protein, 48 g carbohydrate, 4 g dietary fiber, 5 g fat, 1 g saturated fat, 0 mg cholesterol, 32 mg sodium

## CARAMELIZED PEACHES IN SWEET RICOTTA
Serves 8

1½ cups part-skim ricotta cheese
1 teaspoon vanilla extract
3 tablespoons mild honey
½ cup granulated sugar
1 orange, juice and grated peel
1½ tablespoons unsalted butter
2 tablespoons grated ginger root
8 medium-sized ripe peaches, peeled and sliced,
    or 6 cups frozen unsweetened peach slices

2 tablespoons orange-flavored liqueur, optional
fresh mint leaves, as garnish

1. Place ricotta in a food processor and blend until
completely smooth. Remove and stir in vanilla extract
and honey. Refrigerate until ready to serve. (This can
be done ahead—the ricotta will become more honey-
flavored.)

2. When ready to serve, prepare and premeasure all
ingredients and have assembled by skillet. This dish
will cook quickly. Organize dessert bowls or plates.
Mound equal amount of sweetened ricotta cheese on
each plate.

3. Heat a 10-inch skillet over medium-high heat on
the range top. Sprinkle sugar into dry, hot skillet.
Shake pan to distribute sugar evenly on surface of
skillet. Lower heat to medium and allow sugar to melt
and turn caramel-colored (about 10 to 12 minutes).
Do not rush this process or the sugar will burn and
scorch. When sugar is mostly liquid and golden
brown, remove pan from heat. Carefully add, all at
once, the orange juice, peel, butter, and ginger. Cook
and stir until sugar is mostly dissolved. Add peach
slices, return pan to heat, and continue cooking and
gently stirring until peaches are barely done and a
rich, flavorful sauce has been created. Add brandy, if
desired, and cook for about 1 minute.

4. Spoon equal amounts of peaches and sauce over the
mounds of cheese and decorate each with a fresh mint
leaf or sprig of mint. Serve immediately.

**Chef's Notes:** The best hot dessert sauces truly begin with the caramelization of sugar. The rich flavor of the caramel infuses through the butter and fruit flavors to produce an exquisite taste. Although we have used a modest amount of butter, increased amounts are often used. This Ricotta sauce is delicious over fresh berries, bananas, apples, nectarines, etc.

**Nutrition information per serving (not including optional liqueur):** 450 calories, 13 g protein, 79 g carbohydrate, 6 g dietary fiber, 13 g fat, 8 g saturated fat, 45 mg cholesterol, 115 mg sodium

*Recipe developed for the Produce for Better Health Foundation by Carmen I. Jones, CCP. All 5-A-Day recipes meet nutrition standards that maintain fruits and vegetables as healthy foods.*

## PEAR AND APPLE CRISP WITH CRANBERRIES
Serves 8 (1¼ cups each)

- 4 medium almost-ripe pears
- 4 medium crisp apples (my favorite is fuji)
- 1 cup dried cranberries
- 3 tablespoons water
- 1 lemon, juice and grated peel
- 1 cup brown sugar, divided into 2 portions
- 1 teaspoon cardamom, divided into 2 portions
- ½ cup whole rolled oats
- ½ cup all-purpose flour
- 2 tablespoons butter
- 1 cup vanilla yogurt (optional)

1. Preheat the oven to 375°F.

2. Peel the pears and apples, cut into quarters, and core. Cut into large dice and place in lightly greased, shallow baking casserole. Sprinkle evenly with cranberries and water.

3. Sprinkle grated lemon peel over fruit mixture.

4. Combine ½ cup brown sugar with ½ teaspoon cardamom and sprinkle over fruit.

5. Combine rolled oats, flour, and remaining sugar and cardamom in medium bowl. Add butter and work with a fork until mixture is well-blended but crumbly. Add lemon juice and mix thoroughly. Sprinkle evenly over entire fruit mixture. Bake for 45 minutes. Allow the crisp to cool slightly.

6. If desired, stir yogurt in a small bowl until creamy. Top crisp with yogurt.

**Nutrition information per serving (not including optional yogurt):** 290 calories, 0 g protein, 65 g carbohydrate, 5 g dietary fiber, 3.5 g fat, 2 g saturated fat, 10 mg cholesterol, 40 mg sodium

*Recipe developed for the Produce for Better Health Foundation by Carmen I. Jones, CCP. All 5-A-Day recipes meet nutrition standards that maintain fruits and vegetables as healthy foods.*

## YOGURT SMOOTHIE
Serves 1

½ cup light yogurt (approximately 120 calories
per 8 ounce cup), vanilla or the same flavor as
the fruit you're adding
½ cup 1 percent milk
½ cup fresh or frozen fruit (peaches, berries,
banana slices, etc.
sweetener, if desired (e.g. Equal, Splenda, etc.)

1. Combine all ingredients in a blender and blend until light and frothy.

**Nutrition information per serving:** 139 calories, 13 g protein, 23 g
carbohydrate, 2 g fat, 1 g saturated fat, 5 mg cholesterol, 165 mg
sodium, 4 g dietary fiber

## DR. KEITH'S LOW-FAT HOT CHOCOLATE
Serves 1

1 tablespoon cocoa powder (if you like it very
chocolatey, use a rounded tablespoon)
2 packets sweetener (e.g. Equal, Splenda, etc.)
¾ cup water
1⅓ cup nonfat dry milk powder
2 tablespoons nonfat evaporated milk (not
sweetened condensed milk!)

1. Put the cocoa powder and sweetener in a mug.

2. Boil the water and pour it in the mug, stirring constantly until the cocoa powder is dissolved.

3. Slowly add nonfat milk powder, stirring as you go. Then stir in evaporated milk.

**Nutrition information per serving:** 118 calories, 11 g protein, 11 g carbohydrate, 2 g dietary fiber, 1 g fat, .5 g saturated fat, 5 mg cholesterol, 161 mg sodium